Primary Carcinomas of the Liver

Contemporary Issues in Cancer Imaging

A Multidisciplinary Approach

Series Editor

Rodney H. Reznek

Cancer Imaging, St Bartholomew's Hospital, London

Editorial Adviser

Janet E. Husband

Diagnostic Radiology, Royal Marsden Hospital, Surrey

Current titles in the series

Cancer of the Ovary
Lung Cancer
Colorectal Cancer
Carcinoma of the Kidney
Carcinoma of the Esophagus
Carcinoma of the Bladder
Squamous Cell Cancer of the Neck
Prostate Cancer
Interventional Radiological Treatment of Liver Tumors
Pancreatic Cancer
Gastric Cancer

Forthcoming titles in the series

Breast Cancer

Primary Carcinomas of the Liver

Edited by

Hero K. Hussain

Isaac R. Francis

Series Editor

Rodney H. Reznek

Editorial Adviser

Janet E. Husband

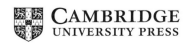

CAMBRIDGE
UNIVERSITY PRESS

CAMBRIDGE UNIVERSITY PRESS
Cambridge, New York, Melbourne, Madrid, Cape Town, Singapore, São Paulo, Delhi

Cambridge University Press
The Edinburgh Building, Cambridge CB2 8RU, UK

Published in the United States of America by Cambridge University Press, New York

www.cambridge.org
Information on this title: www.cambridge.org/9780521519519

First published 2010

Printed in the United Kingdom at the University Press, Cambridge

A catalogue record for this publication is available from the British Library

Library of Congress Cataloguing in Publication data
Primary carcinomas of the liver / edited by Hero K. Hussain and Isaac R. Francis.
    p.   ;   cm. – (Contemporary issues in cancer imaging)
Includes bibliographical references and index.
ISBN 978-0-521-51951-9 (hardback)
1. Liver–Cancer.   I. Hussain, Hero K.   II. Francis, Isaac R.   III. Series: Contemporary issues in cancer imaging.
[DNLM: 1. Carcinoma, Hepatocellular.   2. Cholangiocarcinoma.   WI 735 P9516 2010]
RC280.L5P746   2010
616.99′436 – dc22   2009033909

ISBN 978-0-521-51951-9 Hardback

Contents

Color plates follow page 84.

Contributors

Sharon Bihlmeyer
Department of Pathology
University of Michigan
Ann Arbor, MI
USA

Elaine M. Caoili
Department of Radiology
University of Michigan
Ann Arbor, MI
USA

Isaac R. Francis
Department of Radiology
University of Michigan
Ann Arbor, MI
USA

Orit Gutfeld
Department of Radiation Oncology
University of Michigan
Ann Arbor, MI
USA

Hero K. Hussain
Department of Radiology
University of Michigan
Ann Arbor, MI
USA

Gazala N. Khan
Division of Hematology and Oncology
University of Michigan
Ann Arbor, MI
USA

Edward Kim
Division of Hematology and Oncology
University of Michigan
Ann Arbor, MI
USA

James A. Knol
Department of General Surgery
University of Michigan
Ann Arbor, MI
USA

Venkat N. Krishnamurthy
Department of Radiology
University of Michigan
Ann Arbor, MI
USA

Sean Kumer
Department of Surgery
University of Michigan
Ann Arbor, MI
USA

Peter S. Liu
Department of Radiology
University of Michigan
Ann Arbor, MI
USA

Jorge A. Marrero
Department of Medicine
University of Michigan
Ann Arbor, MI
USA

Barbara McKenna
Department of Pathology
University of Michigan
Ann Arbor, MI
USA

Ajaykumar C. Morani
Department of Radiology
University of Michigan
Ann Arbor, MI
USA

Charlie Pan
Department of Radiation Oncology
University of Michigan
Ann Arbor, MI
USA

Shawn J. Pelletier
Department of General Surgery
University of Michigan
Ann Arbor, MI
USA

Jonathon M. Willatt
Department of Radiology
University of Michigan
Ann Arbor, MI
USA

Mark M. Zalupski
Division of Hematology and Oncology
University of Michigan
Ann Arbor, MI
USA

Series foreword

Imaging has become pivotal in all aspects of the management of patients with cancer. At the same time, it is acknowledged that optimal patient care is best achieved by a multidisciplinary team approach. The explosion of technological developments in imaging over the past years has meant that all members of the multidisciplinary team should understand the potential applications, limitations, and advantages of all the evolving and exciting imaging techniques. Equally, to understand the significance of the imaging findings and to contribute actively to management decisions and to the development of new clinical applications for imaging, it is critical that the radiologist should have sufficient background knowledge of different tumors. Thus the radiologist should understand the pathology, the clinical background, the therapeutic options, and the prognostic indicators of malignancy.

Contemporary Issues in Cancer Imaging – A Multidisciplinary Approach aims to meet the growing requirement for radiologists to have detailed knowledge of the individual tumors about which they are involved in making management decisions. A series of single subject issues, each of which is dedicated to a single tumor site, edited by recognized expert guest editors, include contributions from basic scientists, pathologists, surgeons, oncologists, radiologists, and others.

Although the series is written predominantly for the radiologist, it is hoped that individual issues will contain sufficient varied information so as to be of interest to all medical disciplines and to other health professionals managing patients with cancer. As with imaging, advances have been made in all these disciplines related to cancer management, and it is our fervent hope that this series, bringing together expertise from such a range of related specialties, will not only promote the understanding and rational application of modern imaging but will also help to achieve the ultimate goal of improving outcomes of patients with cancer.

Rodney H. Reznek
London

Preface to Primary Carcinomas of the Liver

The incidence of liver cancer in the United States and worldwide is increasing. The majority of primary liver cancers in the United States are hepatocellular carcinomas (HCC), with cholangiocarcinomas being the next most common. This trend is due to an increase in chronic hepatitis C, which along with hepatitis B is a major risk factor for liver cancer. Other contributing factors include heavy alcohol consumption, fatty liver disease, obesity, diabetes mellitus, and iron storage diseases. Although in general the mortality rates are high, survival rates in some countries are showing some improvement as more patients are being diagnosed with earlier stage tumors by means of aggressive surveillance with serologic tumor markers and diagnostic imaging. Advances in imaging techniques such as diffusion-weighted magnetic resonance imaging (MRI) and positron emission tomography–computed tomography (PET–CT) have helped in improving the detection and characterization of smaller earlier stage tumors. Treatment by means of resection or transplantation has excellent survival rates and, for patients who are not surgical candidates, ablative therapies and transarterial chemoembolization are suitable alternatives. Recently, for advanced HCC, anti-angiogenic agents have been employed with encouraging results. The role of radiotherapy in patients with cholangiocarcinoma and HCC who are poor surgical candidates is increasing.

The purpose of this edition of *Contemporary Issues in Cancer Imaging* is to review the epidemiology, screening, and diagnostic imaging techniques as well as roles of various therapeutic management strategies of common primary hepatic malignancies.

Hero K. Hussain
Isaac R. Francis

Epidemiology of hepatocellular carcinoma and cholangiocarcinoma

Jorge A. Marrero

Hepatocellular carcinoma (HCC) is the fifth most common cancer and the third cause of cancer-related deaths worldwide [1]. Cholangiocarcinoma (CCA) is the second most common primary liver tumor and is less common than HCC. The latest data from the Surveillance, Epidemiology and End Results (SEER) program, a population-based study on cancer incidence, prevalence, and mortality in the United States, show that primary liver cancer (90% HCC and 10% CCA) is one of few tumors with a rising incidence over the last 10 years (Figure 1.1). We herein discuss the epidemiology and risk factors for these tumors.

Hepatocellular carcinoma

The largest concentration of HCC cases in the world is in Asia, followed by Africa, Europe, and North and South America [2]. The incidence of HCC varies among ethnic groups, with increasing incidence rates found in Japanese (5.5/100 000 in men and 4.3/100 000 in women), African American (7.1/100 000 in men and 2.1/100 000 in women), Hispanic (9.8/100 000 in men and 3.5/100 000 in women), and Chinese (16.2/100 000 in men and 5/100 000 in women) populations. Even though the incidence rate is greater in men compared to women, there is a 2- to 5-fold higher incidence rate among women of various ethnicities compared to non-Hispanic white women. During the last two decades, an increasing trend in the incidence of HCC has been noted in Australia, Central Europe, the United Kingdom, Japan, and North America [3]. In addition, there has been an increase in HCC-related mortality in all countries during the same two decades. In the United States, the incidence of HCC has increased in recent years, and the distribution of patients with HCC has shifted toward younger patients, with the greatest increase in those between 45 and 60 years of age, likely due to the aging of the cohort infected with chronic hepatitis C (HCV) during the 1960s and 1970s [4]. The recent review of

Primary Carcinomas of the Liver, ed. Hero K. Hussain and Isaac R. Francis. Published by Cambridge University Press. © Cambridge University Press 2010.

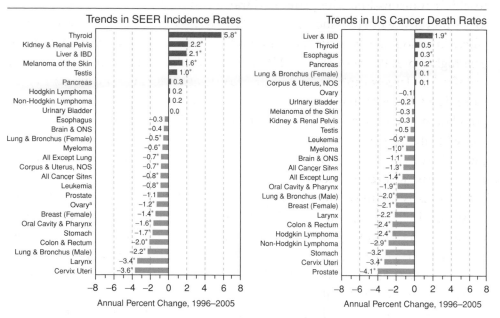

Figure 1.1 Trends in incidence and death rates from 1996 to 2005 based on the Surveillance, Epidemiology and End Results (SEER) program. Primary liver tumors (liver + IBD) account for the third highest increase in incidence and for the highest increase in death rates. Liver = hepatocellular carcinoma; IBD = intrahepatic bile duct cancer or cholangiocarcinoma; ONS = other nervous system; NOS = not otherwise specified.

the SEER program in the United States has shown that over the last 10 years HCC has been the tumor with the highest increase in incidence compared to other solid tumors.

Risk factors

The etiological agents leading to HCC have been largely established. In Japan, Europe, and America in approximately 60% of the patients with HCC, it is attributed to chronic HCV infection, in 20% it is attributed to chronic hepatitis B (HBV) infection, and in 20% it is attributed to cryptogenic and alcoholic liver disease. However, in Asia and Africa more than 80% of patients with HCC have underlying HBV infection [3,5]. The broad traits of the epidemiology of HCC can be traced to the prevalence of hepatotrophic viral infections. Chronic HBV infection is the most common underlying etiology of HCC in the world [6]. In high prevalence areas such as Eastern Asia, China, and Africa, approximately 8% of the population is chronically infected as a result of vertical (mother-to-child) or horizontal (child-to-child) transmission. The pattern of transmission is different in areas with a lower prevalence of HBV such as North America, Western Europe, and Australia, where infection mostly occurs in adulthood through sexual and parenteral routes. The higher prevalence of chronic HBV, as well as the longer period of exposure to infection, largely explains the higher HBV-related HCC risk in endemic areas. Chronic HCV infection is found in a variable proportion of HCC cases in different populations, accounting for 75–90% of cases of HCC in Japan, 31–47% in the United States, 44–76% in Italy, and 60–75% in Spain [6]. HCC is the cancer with the highest increase in incidence rates over the last 10 years in the United States, and the driving force behind this increase is chronic HCV infection [7].

Cirrhosis is the most important risk factor for the development of HCC [8]. As shown in Table 1.1, the risk of HCC increases significantly in patients with cirrhosis. The risk of HCC in persons with HBV-related cirrhosis ranges from 2.2 to 4.3 per 100 person-years, whereas it is less than 1 per 100 person-years in non-cirrhotic patients. It is estimated that approximately 20% of patients with HBV-related HCC present without cirrhosis, indicating that other factors are important in hepatocarcinogenesis. The risk of HCC among patients with chronic HCV infection also occurs in the setting of cirrhosis as shown in Table 1.1. In Japanese studies, the summary incidence rate for HCC was 1.8 per 100 person-years in patients with chronic HCV infection and 7.1 per 100 person-years in persons with compensated cirrhosis. In the United States and Europe, the summary incidence rate was 3.7 per 100 person-years in patients with cirrhosis, which is lower than the rate in Japan.

The natural history of cirrhosis in patients with chronic HCV infection was assessed in 136 patients followed-up for a mean of 6.8 years [9]. The 5-year cumulative risk for HCC was 10%, the mean interval between the diagnosis of cirrhosis and development of HCC was 5 years (range, 0.5–10 years), and the median age for diagnosis of HCC was 63 (range, 50–74). Interestingly, more than half of the patients who developed HCC did not experience hepatic decompensation at the time of HCC diagnosis, indicating that HCC arising in cirrhosis can be clinically silent.

Alcoholic cirrhosis is another well-established major etiologic risk factor for the development of HCC [10]. Recently, an association between non-alcoholic liver disease and HCC has been made [11], but there are no cohort studies evaluating the natural history of non-alcoholic fatty liver disease. Other etiologies of chronic liver

Table 1.1 Incidence rates of HCC in prospective studies in patients with HBV and HCV infection

Setting	Geography	No. of studies	No. of patients	Mean follow-up (y)	HCC incidence[a]
HBV					
Carrier	United States	2	1804	16	0.1
	China	4	18 869	8	0.7
Chronic	Europe	6	471	5.9	0.1
hepatitis	Taiwan	2	461	4	1.0
	Japan	2	737	5.1	0.8
Cirrhosis	Europe	6	401	5.8	2.2
	Taiwan	3	278	4.3	3.2
	Japan	2	306	5.8	4.3
HCV					
Chronic	Europe	1	239	4.2	0.1
hepatitis	Japan	6	1451	6.2	0.8
	Taiwan	1	553	9.2	0.3
Cirrhosis	Europe/United States	13	1284	4.5	3.7
	Japan	7	626	5.8	7.1

[a] Incidence is per 100 person-years. Table modified from [8].

disease such as hemochromatosis, primary biliary cirrhosis, autoimmune hepatitis, and alpha-1 antitrypsin deficiency are less common causes of chronic liver disease with prevalence rates in patients with HCC ranging between 1 and 8% [12,13,14,15]. Improvements in the survival of patients with cirrhosis due to better specialty care may further increase the number of individuals at risk for developing HCC [16].

In addition to the presence of cirrhosis, host and viral factors are important in the process of hepatocarcinogenesis. Host factors including male gender and age greater than 50 years increase the risk for HCC [17]. In persons with chronic HBV infection, evidence of viral replication measured by the antigen status, high serum HBV DNA levels ($>10^5$ copies/mL) [18,19], and HBV genotypes (specifically B) increase the risk of HCC [20]. In contrast, viral factors in chronic HCV infection do not increase the risk of HCC. Other important risk factors in the development of HCC in patients with chronic viral hepatitis are the use of alcohol and tobacco.

Synergism between alcohol and viral hepatitis has been found to increase the risk of HCC [21]. Tobacco is another independent risk factor [22], as is obesity [23]. Aflatoxin B_1 (AFB_1) is a mycotoxin that grows on food stored in humid conditions and is a carcinogen predisposing to human HCC. AFB_1 ingestion has been associated with mutations in the coding regions of p53 tumor suppressor gene [24]. Diabetes has also been shown in prospective studies to increase the risk of HCC [25]. A recent study showed that there is synergy between alcohol exposure greater than 60 g of ethanol per day, greater than 20 pack-years of tobacco smoking, and obesity (body mass > 30 kg/m^2) for increasing the risk of HCC in a predominant population of patients with HCV infection [26]. Therefore, multiple risk factors are important in the process of carcinogenesis in individuals with viral hepatitis.

The burden of HCV-related HCC in the United States is expected to continue to increase during the next decades. A recent study using molecular evolutionary analysis based on the coalescent theory ("molecular clock") investigated the time origin of HCV infection in Japan and the United States [27]. The authors showed an earlier onset of the HCV epidemic in Japan and, therefore, a longer duration of infection in affected individuals, which increases the likelihood for HCC development compared to that in the United States. The authors postulate that the incidence of HCC in the United States will also continue to increase over the next two to three decades. It has been estimated that the number of cases of HCC will continue to increase by 81% (from a baseline of ~13 000/year) by the year 2020, primarily due to the HCV epidemic [28]. This increase may lead to a significant health care burden in North America.

Cholangiocarcinoma

CCA is a neoplasm originating from the intra- or extrahepatic bile duct epithelium [29]. It was not until 1911 that primary liver neoplasms were distinguished based on their cellular origin into "hepatomas" and "cholangiomas" or "hepatocellular carcinomas" and CCA [30,31]. CCA may be considered a rare tumor comprising only 3% of gastrointestinal tumors; however, it is the second most common primary hepatic tumor accounting for 10–15% of primary hepatic malignancies, and its incidence is increasing. Its prevalence is geographically heterogeneous, with the highest rates in Asia, especially Southeast Asia [32]. In Western Europe and the United States, the incidence and mortality of CCA have increased over the last four decades.

In the United States, the age-adjusted incidence of intrahepatic CCA has increased by 165% from 0.32/100 000 (1975–1979) to 0.85/100 000 (1995–1999), with a dramatic increase between 1985 and 1993 [32,33]. An increasing incidence has also been observed in other regions around the globe. Estimated incidence rates in Crete and Greece have increased from 0.998/100 000 (1992–1994) to 3.327/100 000 (1998–2000) [34]. In Japan, the frequency of intrahepatic CCA diagnosed at autopsy increased from 0.31 to 0.58% between 1976–1977 and 1996–1997, respectively [35]. The incidence rates of intrahepatic CCA increased significantly in the United States between 1978 and 2000, with no significant change in the incidence of extrahepatic CCA. The cause of the global increase in the incidence rates for intrahepatic CCA is unclear, and the etiopathogenesis for most patients remains obscure.

Risk factors

The average age at presentation of CCA worldwide is 50 years. In Western nations, most cases of CCA are diagnosed at 65 years of age or older and only rarely before the age of 40 years [32]. In the general population, 52–54% of CCA are observed in male patients; however, mortality data show a higher estimated annual percentage change (EAPC) in women when compared with men with an EAPC of 6.9 ± 1.5 for men and 5.1 ± 1.0 for women [36]. Differences in the prevalence of CCA have been reported globally as well as between different racial and ethnic groups [37]. Globally, the highest prevalence has been described in Southeast Asia. Within the United States, a comparison of the 10-year prevalence between 1990 and 2000 showed a high age-adjusted prevalence of 1.22/100 000 for intrahepatic CCA in Hispanics [38]. Interestingly, within this group, the prevalence was higher in women. The lowest prevalence was described in African Americans, with a prevalence of 0.5/100 000 for men and 0.17/100 000 for women. Asian Pacific Islanders and Caucasians had prevalence rates ranging between these two groups.

In most patients, CCA develops without an identifiable etiology; however, certain risk factors have been established. The most commonly recognized risk factor is primary sclerosing cholangitis. The prevalence of CCA in patients with primary sclerosing cholangitis is 5–15% [39]. The annual incidence rate for CCA in the setting of primary sclerosing cholangitis is 0.6–1.5% [39,40]. Hepatobiliary flukes are another risk factor for CCAs. A strong association has been shown between the species *Opisthorchis viverrini* and *Clonorchis sinensis* and the development of CCA [41] especially in East Asia, which has the highest prevalence of these tumors and where flukes are endemic. These flukes are ingested with undercooked fish and infest the bile ducts and occasionally the gallbladder [42]. Another risk factor for CCA that is also more common in Asian than Western countries is hepatolithiasis. An incidence rate of 10% has been reported in patients with hepatolithiasis [43,44,45]. Additional risk factors for CCA include Caroli's syndrome, congenital hepatic fibrosis, and choledochal cysts, all of which carry a 10–15% increased risk [46,47,48]. The association of intrahepatic CCA with chronic hepatitis C is controversial [49].

In summary, the incidence of both HCC and intrahepatic CCA is rising. The most important feature of HCC is that it occurs in the setting of a chronic liver disease, specifically cirrhosis, with viral hepatitis as the leading cause. Screening or surveillance of this group of patients may improve outcomes. In contrast, there are several risk factors for CCA, but the majority of cases occur without an identifiable risk factor. More studies are needed to identify persons at risk in order to develop screening or surveillance guidelines.

REFERENCES

1. Parkin DM. Global cancer statistics in the year 2000. *Lancet Oncol* 2001; **2**: 533–43.
2. El-Serag HB. Global epidemiology of hepatocellular carcinoma. *Clin Liver Dis* 2001; **5**: 87–107.
3. Bosch FX, Ribes J, Diaz M, and Cleries R. Primary liver cancer: Worldwide incidence and trends. *Gastroenterology* 2004; **127**: S5–S16.
4. El-Serag HB. Hepatocellular carcinoma: Recent trends in the United States. *Gastroenterology* 2004; **127**: S7–S34.
5. Beasley RP, Hwang LY, Lin CC, and Chien CS. Hepatocellular carcinoma and hepatitis B virus: A prospective study of 22,707 men in Taiwan. *Lancet* 1981; **2**: 1129–33.
6. El-Serag HB, Davila JA, Petersen NJ, and McGlynn KA. The continuing increase in the incidence of hepatocellular carcinoma in the United States: An update. *Ann Intern Med* 2003; **139**: 117–23.
7. Davila J, Morgan R, Shaib Y, McGlynn KA, and El-Serag HB. Hepatitis C infection and the rising incidence of hepatocellular carcinoma: A population-based study. *Gastroenterology* 2004; **127**: 1372–80.
8. Fattovich G, Stroffolini T, Zagni I, and Donato F. Hepatocellular carcinoma in cirrhosis: Incidence and risk factors. *Gastroenterology* 2004; **127**: S35–S50.
9. Niederau C, Lange C, Heintges T, *et al.* Prognosis of hepatitis C: Results of a large, prospective cohort study. *Hepatology* 1998; **28**: 1687–95.
10. El Serag HB and Mason AC. Risk factors for the rising rates of primary liver cancer in the United States. *Arch Intern Med* 2000; **160**: 3227–30.
11. Marrero JA, Fontana RJ, Su GL, Conjeevaram HS, Emick DM, and Lok AS. NAFLD may be a common underlying liver disease in patients with hepatocellular carcinoma in the United States. *Hepatology* 2002; **36**: 1349–54.

12. El-Serag HB. Epidemiology of hepatocellular carcinoma. *Clin Liver Dis* 2001; **5**: 87–107.

13. Deugnier Y and Turlin B. Iron and hepatocellular carcinoma. *J Gastroenterol Hepatol* 2001; **16**: 491–4.

14. Farinati F, Floreani A, De Maria N, Fagiuoli S, Naccarato R, and Chiaramonte M. Hepatocellular carcinoma in primary biliary cirrhosis. *J Hepatol* 1994; **21**: 315–16.

15. Nishiyama R, Kanai T, Abe J, *et al.* Hepatocellular carcinoma associated with autoimmune hepatitis. *J Hepatobiliary Pancreat Surg* 2004; **11**: 215–19.

16. Carbonell N, Pauwels A, Serfaty L, Fourdan O, Levy VG, and Poupon R. Improved survival after variceal bleeding in patients with cirrhosis over the past two decades. *Hepatology* 2004; **40**: 652–9.

17. Hassan MM, Frome A, Patt YZ, and El-Serag HB. Rising prevalence of hepatitis C virus infection among patients recently diagnosed with hepatocellular carcinoma in the United States. *J Clin Gastroenterol* 2002; **35**: 266–9.

18. Yang HI, Lu SN, Liaw YF, *et al.* Taiwan Community-Based Cancer Screening Project Group: Hepatitis B e antigen and the risk of hepatocellular carcinoma. *N Engl J Med* 2002; **347**: 168–74.

19. Chen CJ, Yang HI, Su J, *et al.* REVEAL-HBV Study Group: Risk of hepatocellular carcinoma across a biological gradient of serum hepatitis B virus DNA level. *JAMA* 2006; **295**: 65–73.

20. Chan HL, Tse CH, Mo F, *et al.* High viral load and hepatitis B virus subgenotype ce are associated with increased risk of hepatocellular carcinoma. *J Clin Oncol* 2008; **26**: 177–82.

21. Donato F, Tagger A, Gelatti U, *et al.* Alcohol and hepatocellular carcinoma: The effect of lifetime intake and viral hepatitis infection in men and women. *Am J Epidemiol* 2002; **155**: 323–31.

22. El-Serag HB, Marrero JA, Rudolph L, and Reddy KR. Diagnosis and treatment of hepatocellular carcinoma. *Gastroenterology* 2008; **134**: 1752–63.

23. Calle EE, Rodriguez C, Walker-Thurmond K, and Thun MJ. Overweight, obesity, and mortality from cancer in a prospectively studied cohort of U.S. adults. *N Engl J Med* 2003; **348**: 1625–38.

24. Wang LY, Hatch M, Chen CJ, *et al.* Aflatoxin exposure and risk of hepatocellular carcinoma in Taiwan. *Int J Cancer* 1996; **67**: 620–5.

25. El-Serag HB, Tran T, and Everhart JE. Diabetes increases the risk of chronic liver disease and hepatocellular carcinoma. *Gastroenterology* 2004; **126**: 460–8.

26. Marrero JA, Fontana RJ, Fu S, Conjeevaram HS, Su GL, and Lok AS. Alcohol, tobacco and obesity are synergistic risk factors for hepatocellular carcinoma. *J Hepatol* 2005; **42**: 218–24.

27. Tanaka Y, Hanada K, Mizokami M, *et al.* Inaugural Article: A comparison of the molecular clock of hepatitis C virus in the United States and Japan predicts that hepatocellular carcinoma incidence in the United States will increase over the next two decades. *Proc Natl Acad Sci U S A* 2002; **99**: 15584–9.

28. Singal A and Marrero JA. Screening for hepatocellular carcinoma. *Gastroenterol Hepatol* 2008; **4**: 201–8.

29. de Groen PC, Gores GJ, LaRusso NF, *et al.* Biliary tract cancers. *N Engl J Med* 1999; **341**: 1368–78.

30. Goldzieher M and von Bokay Z. Der primaere leberkrebs. *Virchows Arch* 1911; **203**: 75–131.

31. Klatskin G. Adenocarcinoma of the hepatic duct at its bifurcation within the porta hepatis: An unusual tumor with distinctive clinical and pathological features. *Am J Med* 1965; **38**: 241–56.

32. Patel T. Increasing incidence and mortality of primary intrahepatic cholangiocarcinoma in the United States. *Hepatology* 2001; **33**: 1353–7.

33. Shaib YH, Davila JA, McGlynn K, *et al.* Rising incidence of intrahepatic cholangiocarcinoma in the United States: A true increase? *J Hepatol* 2004; **40**: 472–7.

34. Mouzas IA, Dimoulios P, Vlachonikolis IG, Skordilis P, Zoras O, and Kouroumalis E. Increasing incidence of cholangiocarcinoma in Crete 1992–2000. *Anticancer Res* 2002; **22**: 3637–41.

35. Okuda K, Nakanuma Y, and Miyazaki M. Cholangiocarcinoma: Recent progress. Part 1. Epidemiology and etiology. *J Gastroenterol Hepatol* 2002; **17**: 1049–55.

36. Welzel TM, McGlynn KA, Hsing AW, *et al.* Impact of classification of hilar cholangiocarcinoma (Klatskin tumors) on the incidence of intra- and extrahepatic cholangiocarcinoma in the United States. *J Natl Cancer Inst* 2006; **98**: 873–5.

37. Patel T. Worldwide trends in mortality from biliary tract malignancies. *BMC Cancer* 2002; **2**: 1–5.

38. McLean L and Patel T. Racial and ethnic variations in the epidemiology of intrahepatic cholangiocarcinoma in the United States. *Liver Int* 2006; **26**: 1047–53.

39. Burak K, Angulo P, Pasha TM, Egan K, Petz J, and Lindor KD. Incidence and risk factors for cholangiocarcinoma in primary sclerosing cholangitis. *Am J Gastroenterol* 2004; **99**: 523–6.

40. Bergquist A, Ekbom A, Olsson R, *et al.* Hepatic and extrahepatic malignancies in primary sclerosing cholangitis. *J Hepatol* 2002; **36**: 321–7.

41. Watanapa P and Watanapa WB. Liver fluke-associated cholangiocarcinoma. *Br J Surg* 2002; **89**: 962–70.

42. Kurathong S, Lerdverasirikul P, Wongpaitoon V, *et al.* Opisthorchis viverrini infection and cholangiocarcinoma: A prospective, case-controlled study. *Gastroenterology* 1985; **89**: 151–6.

43. Kubo S, Kinoshita H, Hirohashi K, *et al.* Hepatolithiasis associated with cholangiocarcinoma. *World J Surg* 1995; **19**: 637–41.

44. Lesurtel M, Regimbeau JM, Farges O, Colombat M, Sauvanet A, and Belghiti J. Intrahepatic cholangiocarcinoma and hepatolithiasis: An unusual association in Western countries. *Eur J Gastroenterol Hepatol* 2002; **14**: 1025–7.

45. Su CH, Shyr YM, Lui WY, *et al.* Hepatolithiasis associated with cholangiocarcinoma. *Br J Surg* 1997; **84**: 969–73.

46. Chapman RW. Risk factors for biliary tract carcinogenesis. *Ann Oncol* 1999; **10**: S308–S311.

47. Lipsett PA, Pitt HA, Colombani PM, *et al.* Choledochal cyst disease: A changing pattern of presentation. *Ann Surg* 1994; **220**: 644–52.

48. Scott J, Shousha S, Thomas HC, *et al.* Bile duct carcinoma: A late complication of congenital hepatic fibrosis. Case report and review of literature. *Am J Gastroenterol* 1980; **73**: 113–19.

49. Change KY, Chang JY, Yen Y. Increasing incidence of intrahepatic cholangiocarcinoma and its relationship to chronic viral hepatitis. *J Natl Compr Canc Netw* 2009; **7**: 423–7.

2

Surveillance and screening for hepatocellular carcinoma

Jorge A. Marrero and Hero K. Hussain

The decision to screen an at-risk population for cancer is based on well-established criteria [1]. Although the overall goal is to reduce morbidity and mortality from cancer, the objective of screening is to use a relatively simple and inexpensive test in a large number of individuals to determine whether they are likely or unlikely to have the cancer for which they are being screened [2]. Screening is the one-time application of a test that allows detection of preclinical tumors, tumors at an early stage when they are asymptomatic with no clinical suspicion, and when curative intervention may achieve the goal of reducing morbidity and mortality. Surveillance is the continuous monitoring of disease occurrence (using the screening test) within a population to accomplish the same goals of screening [3]. Criteria have been developed, first promoted by the World Health Organization, to assess the benefits of screening for a specific disease [4]. This review will evaluate the process of screening/surveillance for hepatocellular carcinoma (HCC).

Cirrhosis has been recognized as the most important risk factor for the development of HCC [3]. Hepatitis C (HCV) and hepatitis B (HBV) are the major etiological agents that lead to the development of HCC [5]. HCV-associated cirrhosis is the causative agent that has been largely responsible for the increase in incidence of HCC in the United States. However, HBV is the leading cause of HCC worldwide, particularly in Asia and Africa. Therefore, there is a target population to which surveillance tests can be applied. Table 2.1 shows the recommendations for surveillance in patients with cirrhosis.

For surveillance to be effective, excellent treatment for early-stage tumors should be available. For early-stage tumors, surgical resection has provided 5-year survival rates of 70% in carefully selected patients with single small asymptomatic tumors (<5 cm in maximal diameter) preserved hepatic function and no evidence of portal hypertension [6]. Liver transplantation is the preferred method of treatment for patients not amenable to surgical resection but with tumors restricted to the

Primary Carcinomas of the Liver, ed. Hero K. Hussain and Isaac R. Francis. Published by Cambridge University Press. © Cambridge University Press 2010.

Table 2.1 AASLD recommendations for the surveillance for HCC in patients with cirrhosis

Recommendation	Levels of evidence[a]
Surveillance for HCC should be performed using ultrasonography	II
AFP alone should not be used for screening unless ultrasound is not available	II
Patients should be screened at 6- to 12-month intervals	II
The surveillance interval does not need to be shortened for patients at higher risk of HCC	III

[a] Levels of evidence from I (highest) to III (lowest) [5]. AASLD, American Association for the Study of Liver Diseases.

Milan criteria (single nodule ≤5 cm or up to three nodules each ≤3 cm in diameter) [7]. The 5-year survival reported for liver transplantation is 74% [5]. Ablative treatments, specifically percutaneous ethanol injection and radiofrequency ablation, have 5-year survival rates of more than 37% in Barcelona Clinic Liver Cancer (BCLC) stage A patients not amenable to resection or transplantation [5]. Thus, therapies that result in excellent 5-year survival exist for patients with early-stage HCC, and an efficacious surveillance program is therefore critical for the identification of early-stage HCC.

The ideal surveillance test should be specific for preclinical HCC in the cirrhotic liver, regardless of the etiology of cirrhosis. It should be easily measurable, reproducible, minimally invasive, and acceptable to patients and physicians [8]. Both radiographic and serologic tests are currently used for HCC surveillance.

Ultrasound has been recommended as the primary radiologic screening test for HCC [5]. It is the least expensive, non-invasive, and widely available, which makes it an attractive screening test. To date, there has been no randomized controlled trial in patients with cirrhosis to assess the efficacy of ultrasound as a screening test, and its performance has been evaluated primarily in retrospective cohort studies as shown in Table 2.2 [9,10,11,12,13,14,15]. The reported sensitivities of ultrasound for the detection of early-stage HCC range from 29% to 100%, and the specificities range from 94% to 100%. The high degree of operator dependence and differences in equipment and body habitus are significant limitations that preclude it from being the optimal imaging surveillance test for HCC.

Table 2.2 Performance of ultrasonography as a surveillance test for HCC

Author	Cohort	No. early HCC cases	Sensitivity/specificity (%/%)
Pateron *et al.* [9]	Childs A – B	14	29/96
Bolondi *et al.* [10]	Childs A – B	61	82/95
Tong *et al.* [11]	Child A	31	54/89
Cottone *et al.* [12]	Childs A	5	80/100
Kobayashi *et al.* [13]	Cirrhosis[a]	8	50/98
Sheu *et al.* [14]	Cirrhosis[a]	7	100/100
Oka *et al.* [15]	Cirrhosis[a]	40	68/NA

[a] The population of cirrhosis was not specified further. NA, not available.

Alpha-fetoprotein (AFP) has been the most widely used serologic test to screen for HCC. The operating characteristics of AFP are dependent on the cutoff level chosen to support the diagnosis of HCC. At higher cutoff levels, the test is more specific for HCC but at a cost of decreased sensitivity; at low cutoff levels, conversely, AFP becomes increasingly sensitive but with a higher rate of false positives [16]. A case–control study of 170 patients with HCC, of whom 60% had advanced HCC, and 170 matched patients without HCC demonstrated that the optimal cutoff was 20 ng/mL using receiver operating curve (ROC) analysis [17]. Therefore, a level greater than 20 ng/mL is the most commonly used cutoff in clinical practice to trigger a recall test for the diagnosis of HCC. A recent systematic review of five studies evaluating AFP greater than 20 ng/mL for the detection of HCC in patients with HCV-related cirrhosis showed sensitivities ranging from 41 to 65% and specificities ranging from 80 to 94% [18]. In addition, serum AFP values are frequently elevated among patients with chronic HCV with advanced hepatic fibrosis even in the absence of HCC, with the levels declining after antiviral therapy [19]. Better tests are needed to improve the detection of early-stage HCC.

The most reliable method to evaluate the efficacy of ultrasound and AFP for HCC surveillance would be a randomized controlled trial. There have been two large randomized controlled trials conducted in China using ultrasound and AFP among patients with chronic HBV [20,21]. In both trials, surveillance was conducted every 6 months and compared to patients who did not receive any routine screening. The first study evaluated 17 920 patients who were carriers of HBV; they were randomized to either surveillance ($n = 8109$) or no surveillance ($n = 9711$) and were followed up for an average of 14.4 months [20]. Of the patients randomized to the surveillance group, 38 had had HCC; 76.8% of whom were at a subclinical stage, and 70.6% of those underwent resection. In the non-surveillance group, 18 patients had HCC, and none could undergo resection due to advanced disease ($p < 0.01$). Accordingly, the 1-year and 2-year survival rates for the surveillance group were 88.1% and 77.5%, respectively, compared to none more than 1 year for the non-surveillance group. The second randomized controlled trial evaluated 19 200 HBV carriers who were randomized to either surveillance ($n = 9757$) or no surveillance ($n = 9443$) [21]. A total of 86 patients developed HCC in the surveillance group, of which 45% were early stage, compared to 67 patients with HCC in the no surveillance group, of which none were early stage. The mortality rate of patients undergoing surveillance was significantly lower than that of patients in the control group [83.2 vs. 131.5 per 100 000, ($p < 0.01$), with a hazard ratio of 0.63 (95% confidence interval, .41–.98)]. These results demonstrate that the strategy of surveillance among patients with chronic HBV reduces overall mortality. The main problem with both studies is that they did not mention the number of patients who had cirrhosis or evidence of viral replication who are at the highest risk for developing HCC, and most likely both studies included patients who were asymptomatic carriers, who are at a lower risk for developing HCC. Therefore, the results are not generalizable to the majority of patients at risk for developing HCC.

Although randomized controlled trials have been performed in China on patients with chronic HBV, the results cannot be extrapolated to cirrhotic patients, who account for the majority of patients with HCC worldwide. No randomized trials have been performed in a cirrhotic population, so most of the data on surveillance in patients with cirrhosis come from cohort studies. The results of these studies are also fraught with lead-time and length-time biases that limit their generalizability with regard to improvement of survival with surveillance. The early-stage detection rate has ranged between 24 and 91% [22,23,24,25,26]. Therefore, the impact of surveillance on mortality in patients with cirrhosis has been assessed in only non-randomized trials to date.

Surveillance for any tumor should be cost effective. The standard threshold for cost-effectiveness has been determined to be a maximum of $50 000 per quality-adjusted life year (QALY). Economic models studying the benefits of surveillance programs in HCC have been developed. Surveillance with biannual AFP and ultra-sonography in Child-Pugh Class A cirrhotics increases the mean life expectancy with cost-effectiveness ratios between $26 000 and $55 000 per QALY [27]. When a similar analysis was performed in HCV cirrhotics, the cost–utility ratio was $26 689 per QALY [28]. Therefore, screening with ultrasonography and AFP has been shown to be cost-effective in compensated cirrhotics. Other imaging modalities, such as computed tomography (CT) and magnetic resonance imaging (MRI), are more suitable as diagnostic rather than surveillance tests due to issues such as expense, availability and reproducibility (for MRI), and exposure to ionizing radiation (for CT).

In summary, HCC meets all the World Health Organization criteria for establishing a surveillance program. The current strategy of surveillance with AFP and ultrasonography has been shown in two large randomized controlled trials to reduce mortality in patients with chronic HBV. Although the impact of surveillance in patients with cirrhosis has not been evaluated by a randomized controlled trial, several non-randomized and uncontrolled cohort studies suggest that surveillance can lead to a portion of patients being diagnosed at early stages of disease, and that it is cost-effective.

REFERENCES

1. Cole P and Morrison AS. Basic issues in population screening for cancer. *J Natl Cancer Inst* 1980; **64**: 1263–72.
2. Smith RA. Screening fundamentals. *J Natl Cancer Inst Monogr* 1997: 15–19.
3. Collier J and Sherman M. Screening for hepatocellular carcinoma. *Hepatology* 1998; **27**: 273–8.
4. Meissner HI, Smith RA, Rimer BK, *et al.* Promoting cancer screening: Learning from experience. *Cancer* 2004; **101**: 1107–17.
5. Bruix J and Sherman M. Management of hepatocellular carcinoma. *Hepatology* 2005; **42**: 1208–36.
6. Llovet JM and Bruix J. Early diagnosis and treatment of hepatocellular carcinoma. *Baillieres Best Pract Res Clin Gastroenterol* 2000; **14**: 991–1008.
7. Mazzaferro V, Regalia E, Doci R, *et al.* Liver transplantation for the treatment of small hepatocellular carcinomas in patients with cirrhosis. *N Engl J Med* 1996; **334**: 693–9.
8. Srinivas PR, Kramer BS, and Srivastava S. Trends in biomarker research for cancer detection. *Lancet Oncol* 2001; **2**: 698–704.
9. Pateron D, Ganne N, Trinchet JC, *et al.* Prospective study of screening for hepatocellular carcinoma in Caucasian patients with cirrhosis. *J Hepatol* 1994; **20**: 65–71.
10. Bolondi L, Sofia S, Siringo S, *et al.* Surveillance programme of cirrhotic patients for early diagnosis and treatment of hepatocellular carcinoma: A cost effectiveness analysis. *Gut* 2001; **48**: 251–9.
11. Tong MJ, Blatt LM, and Kao VW. Surveillance for hepatocellular carcinoma in patients with chronic viral hepatitis in the United States of America. *J Gastroenterol Hepatol* 2001; **16**: 553–9.
12. Cottone M, Turri M, Caltagirone M, *et al.* Early detection of hepatocellular carcinoma associated with cirrhosis by ultrasound and alfafetoprotein: A prospective study. *Hepato-Gastroenterology* 1988; **35**: 101–3.

13. Kobayashi K, Sugimoto T, Makino H, *et al.* Screening methods for early detection of hepatocellular carcinoma. *Hepatology* 1985; **5**: 1100–5.

14. Sheu JC, Sung JL, Chen DS, *et al.* Early detection of hepatocellular carcinoma by real-time ultrasonography. A prospective study. *Cancer* 1985; **56**: 660–6.

15. Oka H, Kurioka N, Kim K, *et al.* Prospective study of early detection of hepatocellular carcinoma in patients with cirrhosis. *Hepatology* 1990; **12**: 680–7.

16. Colli A, Fraquelli M, and Conte D. Alpha-fetoprotein and hepatocellular carcinoma. *Am J Gastroenterol* 2006; **101**: 1939.

17. Trevisani F, D'Intino PE, Morselli-Labate AM, *et al.* Serum alpha-fetoprotein for diagnosis of hepatocellular carcinoma in patients with chronic liver disease: Influence of HBsAg and anti-HCV status. *J Hepatol* 2001; **34**: 570–5.

18. Gupta S, Bent S, and Kohlwes J. Test characteristics of alpha-fetoprotein for detecting hepatocellular carcinoma in patients with hepatitis C. A systematic review and critical analysis. *Ann Intern Med* 2003; **139**: 46–50.

19. Di Bisceglie AM, Sterling RK, Chung RT, *et al.* Serum alpha-fetoprotein levels in patients with advanced hepatitis C: Results from the HALT-C Trial. *J Hepatol* 2005; **43**: 434–41.

20. Yang B, Zhang B, Xu Y, *et al.* Prospective study of early detection for primary liver cancer. *J Cancer Res Clin Oncol* 1997; **123**: 357–60.

21. Zhang BH, Yang BH, and Tang ZY. Randomized controlled trial of screening for hepatocellular carcinoma. *J Cancer Res Clin Oncol* 2004; **130**: 417–22.

22. Sangiovanni A, Del Ninno E, Fasani P, *et al.* Increased survival of cirrhotic patients with a hepatocellular carcinoma detected during surveillance. *Gastroenterology* 2004; **126**: 1005–14.

23. Santagostino E, Colombo M, Rivi M, *et al.* A 6-month versus a 12-month surveillance for hepatocellular carcinoma in 559 hemophiliacs infected with the hepatitis C virus. *Blood* 2003; **102**: 78–82.

24. Zoli M, Magalotti D, Bianchi G, Gueli C, Marchesini G, and Pisi E. Efficacy of a surveillance program for early detection of hepatocellular carcinoma. *Cancer* 1996; **78**: 977–85.

25. Tradati F, Colombo M, Mannucci PM, *et al.* A prospective multicenter study of hepatocellular carcinoma in Italian hemophiliacs with chronic hepatitis C. The Study Group of the Association of Italian Hemophilia Centers. *Blood* 1998; **91**: 1173–7.

26. Colombo M, de Franchis R, Del Ninno E, *et al.* Hepatocellular carcinoma in Italian patients with cirrhosis. *N Engl J Med* 1991; **325**: 675–80.

27. Sarasin FP, Giostra E, and Hadengue A. Cost-effectiveness of screening for detection of small hepatocellular carcinoma in western patients with Child-Pugh Class A cirrhosis. *Am J Med* 1996; **101**: 422–34.

28. Arguedas MR, Chen VK, Eloubeidi MA, and Fallon MB. Screening for hepatocellular carcinoma in patients with hepatitis C cirrhosis: a cost-utility analysis. *Am J Gastroenterol* 2003; **98**: 679–90.

3

Pathology of hepatocellular carcinoma, cholangiocarcinoma, and combined hepatocellular-cholangiocarcinoma

Barbara McKenna and Sharon Bihlmeyer

As with any organ or organ system, the liver is the site of a wide variety of neoplasms, both benign and malignant. Overall, the most common primary neoplasm in the liver is the hemangioma, a benign vascular neoplasm that rarely causes diagnostic difficulty [1]. Primary malignant neoplasms include hepatocellular carcinoma (HCC), cholangiocarcinoma (CCA), sarcomas, and an assortment of rare tumors of other types. In adults, the two most common primary malignant tumors are HCC and CCA. Some tumors are mixtures of the two [1]. These two common malignancies will be the topics of the following discussion.

Hepatocellular carcinoma

HCC is a malignant tumor of hepatocytes occurring most commonly in older adults, and is associated with several etiologic factors, including hepatitis B and C, and cirrhosis resulting from steatohepatitis, hemochromatosis, and other causes [2]. Pathologic evaluation of HCC may occur as part of an initial diagnosis when a liver biopsy or fine-needle aspiration (FNA) may yield limited material for study, or when tumors are resected.

Macroscopic features

HCC are typically present within cirrhotic livers, in which they develop fibrous capsules and fibrous intratumoral septae as they enlarge, giving them a firm consistency. Necrosis and intratumoral hemorrhage may be present (Figure 3.1). Satellite nodules may be present at the periphery of large tumors. In non-cirrhotic livers, HCC tends to be softer and unencapsulated. Although one large mass is characteristic, some patients present with several or multiple masses throughout the liver. Multiple small HCC may be difficult to distinguish from nodules of cirrhosis. Rare

Primary Carcinomas of the Liver, ed. Hero K. Hussain and Isaac R. Francis. Published by Cambridge University Press. © Cambridge University Press 2010.

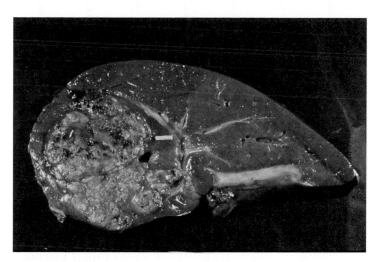

Figure 3.1 HCC (*white line*) in a non-cirrhotic liver. Tumor varies from firm and pale to necrotic and hemorrhagic. (See color plate section.)

examples of HCC, usually in females, are pedunculated. These pedunculated HCC are thought to develop in accessory lobes of liver, and are associated with excellent prognoses after being resected [1,2].

Venous invasion is a characteristic feature of HCC, especially large tumors. Portal and hepatic veins, as well as the vena cava, may be invaded. Tumors smaller than 2 cm rarely have venous invasion, which is considered to be the mechanism of intrahepatic metastasis. Bile duct invasion is uncommon, but does occur in a small percentage of cases [1,2].

Microscopic features

The histologic diagnosis of HCC depends on the identification of hepatocellular differentiation in a neoplasm that also has malignant features. Either criterion may be challenging to satisfy in a given example, because there is great heterogeneity in both the cytologic and architectural features of HCC.

Hepatocellular differentiation is recognized morphologically in neoplastic cells that have a fairly abundant, finely granular eosinophilic cytoplasm and round-to-oval central nuclei with prominent nucleoli and sometimes intranuclear cytoplasmic invaginations.

The cytoplasm may contain any of a number of components that are sometimes seen in non-neoplastic hepatocytes. Cytoplasmic fat droplets may be present, especially in small HCC, and are not necessarily associated with steatosis or steatohepatitis in the surrounding liver parenchyma. Cytoplasmic glycogen, when abundant, may impart a clear appearance to the cytoplasm, requiring distinction from other clear cell tumors such as metastatic renal cell carcinoma of clear cell type. Cells with Mallory's hyaline are present in as many as 20% of HCC, may be numerous, and may be associated with a neutrophilic inflammatory response [1]. Alpha-1 antitrypsin globules appear as round, eosinophilic cytoplasmic globules that are also PAS (periodic acid–Schiff) positive. Large, pale cytoplasmic inclusions resembling the ground glass appearance of cells that contain hepatitis B surface antigen may be present; these inclusions are aggregates of fibrinogen. Architectural similarities to non-neoplastic liver are also useful as evidence of hepatocellular differentiation. Like those of normal liver, the cells of HCC are often arranged in cords that are separated by endothelium-lined, sinusoid-like vascular spaces. Bile canaliculi may be formed by hepatocytes and may either be inconspicuous without special stains (as in normal liver) or dilated with or without luminal bile [1,2].

Malignant features in HCC may be subtle or obvious. In well-differentiated HCC, subtle evidence of malignancy may be found in a slightly increased ratio of nuclear to cytoplasmic volume, macronucleoli, rare mitoses, and the presence of pseudoglandular arrangements of hepatocytes. In poorly differentiated or high-grade HCC, malignancy is obvious, based on classic features of malignancy: nuclear hyperchromasia and pleomorphism, frequent mitoses, the presence of necrosis, and invasion of adjacent tissue. In such cases it may be difficult to find convincing evidence of hepatocellular differentiation [1,2].

Immunohistochemical evidence of hepatocellular differentiation, and of neoplasia, may be employed in challenging cases, as discussed later in this chapter.

Morphologic patterns of hepatocellular carcinoma

The World Health Organization recognizes several patterns of HCC. With a few exceptions, however, these patterns are not of much clinical significance. Mixtures of patterns may be present.

The **trabecular pattern** of HCC is the most common. Cords of tumor cells are of varying widths, generally greater than the two- to three-cell width of hepatocyte cords in normal liver. These cords of tumor cells are separated by sinusoid-like spaces lined by endothelial cells (Figure 3.2). These sinusoid-like spaces are often ectatic, and may become quite dilated in some cases. Dilated bile canaliculi creating pseudoglandular spaces may be present within thickened cords. The supporting stroma lacks the desmoplasia that is common in many other types of carcinoma [2].

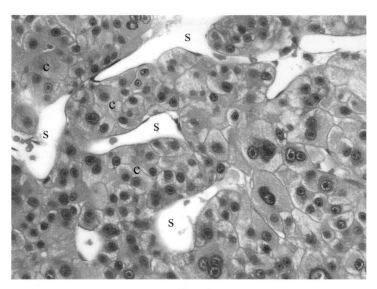

Figure 3.2 The trabecular pattern of HCC is characterized by cords of neoplastic hepatocytes (c) separated by sinusoid-like vascular spaces (s). The neoplasms differ from benign liver cells in having cells with increased ratios of nuclear-to-cytoplasmic volumes and enlarged nuclei with macronucleoli, and by having broader trabeculae. (hematoxylin and eosin [H&E], ×200) (See color plate section.)

Cases of HCC that are dominated by glandlike spaces constitute the **pseudo-glandular** or **acinar pattern** (Figure 3.3). The glandlike spaces are formed mostly by dilated bile canaliculi surrounded by tumor cells, and may contain bile or pro-teinaceous, eosinophilic, PAS-positive material. The **compact pattern** results from compression of the sinusoid-like spaces by tumor cells, giving a solid appearance.

Uncommon examples of HCC that have abundant stromal fibrosis are referred to as **scirrhous HCC**. This HCC variant has fibrous tissue diffusely present along the sinusoid-like vascular spaces, associated with variable atrophy of tumor trabeculae or nests (Figure 3.4). Scirrhous HCC is reported to constitute from 0.2 to 4.6% of cases of HCC, depending on the study [2]. There does not seem to be any difference in age, gender, presence of cirrhosis, association with hepatitis B or C, serum alpha-fetoprotein levels, or stage between scirrhous HCC and other patterns. Interestingly, scirrhous HCC typically occur immediately beneath the capsule or protrude from the surface, and when multiple HCC are present, only those beneath the capsule may have the scirrhous pattern. Due to the abundant fibrosis, these tumors are firm, white, lobulated, and well-circumscribed, and may be misdiagnosed as CCA or mixed hepatocellular-CCA, based on imaging studies. In addition to the stromal fibrosis, these tumors have less hemorrhage and necrosis, more intratumoral portal

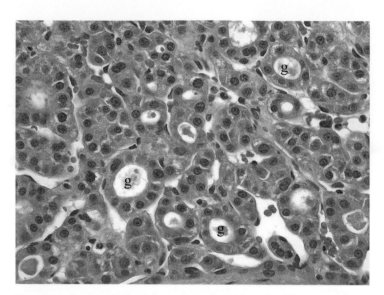

Figure 3.3 The pseudoglandular pattern of HCC has glandlike spaces that are dilated bile canaliculi between neoplastic hepatocytes (g). Many of these spaces contain inspissated bile. (H&E, ×200) (See color plate section.)

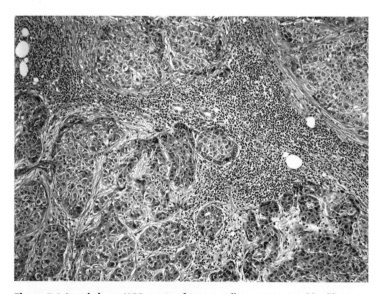

Figure 3.4 In scirrhous HCC, nests of tumor cells are separated by fibrous stroma, often containing a prominent lymphocytic infiltrate. (H&E, ×100) (See color plate section.)

tracts, more clear cell change, more frequent lymphocytic infiltration, and more Mallory's hyaline. The tumor cells are much like those in other patterns of HCC, but are compressed into atrophic cords or nests by the fibrosis. The importance of this HCC variant is threefold. First, its fibrous stroma may result in misdiagnosis

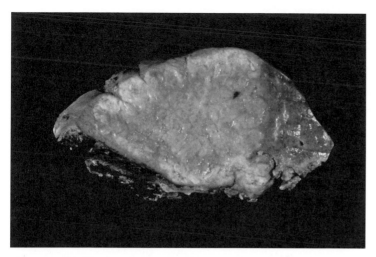

Figure 3.5 This fibrolamellar variant of HCC is present immediately beneath the capsular surface. The tumor is paler than the adjacent red-brown normal parenchyma, and has multiple, white fibrous bands that traverse the mass. (See color plate section.)

based on medical imaging. Second, the abundant stroma may cause histologic confusion with CCA or metastatic adenocarcinoma, complicated by the fact that this scirrhous HCC is more likely to be immunohistochemically cytokeratin 7 positive and hepatocyte paraffin 1 (Hep Par 1) negative, unlike most HCC (see immunohistochemistry discussion later in this chapter). Third and finally, scirrhous HCC are reported to have better prognoses, stage for stage, than other patterns of HCC [3,4].

The **fibrolamellar pattern of HCC** stands apart from all other patterns, because it has different demographic and disease associations and different clinical behavior. Fibrolamellar HCC generally occurs in non-cirrhotic livers in adolescents or young adults. They are rare in Asia and Africa, but more common in Europe and North America. Fibrolamellar HCC presents as a single mass, more often in the left lobe, characterized by a dense central scar from which fibrous septae divide the tumor into lobules (Figure 3.5). These tumors are quite firm and may have central calcification. Microscopically, thick lamellae of hyalinized collagen separate tumor nests or individual tumor cells. The stroma may contain large, thick-walled arteries. The tumor cells are larger than normal hepatocytes, and have abundant, coarsely granular cytoplasm due to the presence of numerous mitochondria. Nuclei are large and vesicular and have prominent nucleoli, but mitoses are rare. Like other HCC, tumor cells may contain fat, alpha-1 antitrypsin globules, pale bodies composed of fibrinogen, or Mallory's hyaline. All series have reported survival periods substantially longer than other HCC after resection [1,2].

Grading of hepatocellular carcinoma

Grading systems for HCC are based primarily on nuclear features. Grade thus defined has been shown to have some correlation with prognosis in large series. However, grading of HCC is not widely used, because it has little prognostic or management significance in individual cases [2].

Immunohistochemical study in the biopsy diagnosis of hepatocellular carcinoma

Most cases of HCC are readily diagnosed based on microscopic examination without the need for special stains, because both criteria of hepatocellular differentiation and malignancy can be readily established morphologically. However, cases that are either exceptionally well or exceptionally poorly differentiated may be more difficult, the former because they are hard to recognize as malignant and the latter because they are hard to recognize as hepatocellular. In particular, needle biopsies of hepatic masses frequently obtain more benign than lesional tissue, and are quite challenging. Immunohistochemical stains may be useful in these two circumstances, with different stains employed depending on which criterion one is trying to satisfy.

The differential diagnosis for well-differentiated carcinoma includes benign cirrhotic nodule, focal nodular hyperplasia, and liver cell adenoma. Because the latter two items have characteristic clinical presentations, the distinction of well-differentiated HCC from benign cirrhotic liver parenchyma is the more common problem. Two immunohistochemical strategies are employed in this differential diagnosis. The first takes advantage of the fact that the endothelial cells that line the sinusoid-like spaces in HCC are different from those in benign liver. In the normal liver, the endothelial cells lining sinusoids are of a special type, different than those in the rest of the body. They do not produce basement membrane material, including the components **laminin** and **type IV collagen**, and they do not mark with antibodies to **CD34**. The CD34 protein is a member of a family of transmembrane sialomucin proteins that are expressed on early hematopoietic and vascular tissue. Little is known about its function. In contrast, the endothelial cells of HCC lack such specialization, and so produce basement membrane components and are marked with anti-CD34 antibodies (Figure 3.6). Thus, sinusoidal staining with immunohistochemical markers for CD34, laminin, or collagen IV have been used to separate HCC from non-neoplastic liver lesions, such as cirrhotic nodules and focal nodular hyperplasia. Of these, CD34 is the most commonly used. Some HCC will have only

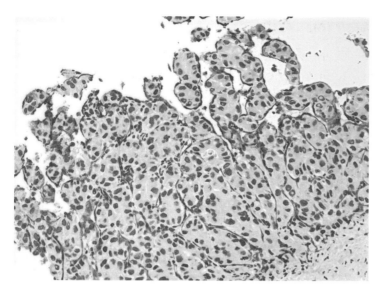

Figure 3.6 The endothelial cells lining the sinusoid-like spaces in HCC are often immunohistochemically positive with antibodies to CD34 (*brown stain* along the edges of tumor cells), unlike normal liver, which lacks such CD34 expression along sinusoids. (CD34 immunohistochemical stain, ×200) (See color plate section.)

patchy CD34 positivity, so this immunohistochemical stain will not solve this problem in all cases, especially in small samples like needle biopsies and FNA specimens. A new antibody that is showing promise in the diagnosis of well-differentiated HCC is **glypican-3**. Glypican-3 is a glycosylphosphatidylinositol anchored membrane protein that is expressed in HCC as well as in hepatoblastoma, melanoma, testicular germ cell tumors, and Wilms' tumor. It is not expressed in normal adult tissues, including normal liver cells. Its sensitivity in identifying HCC is reported to be in the range of 77–88%, with a specificity virtually of 100% in distinguishing well-differentiated HCC from benign liver cell lesions, because it is uniformly negative in normal liver, adenomas, cirrhotic liver, and focal nodular hyperplasia. Some high-grade dysplastic nodules have been reported to express glypican-3 [5,6,7].

A poorly differentiated HCC may be difficult to distinguish from other carcinomas, primary and metastatic. In such cases, malignancy is readily apparent, but hepatocellular differentiation may be difficult to establish. Immunohistochemical strategies to identify hepatocellular differentiation use polyclonal CEA (pCEA), CD10, and Hep Par 1 (and Hepatocyte) antibodies. Hep Par 1 and Hepatocyte are two closely related antibodies that recognize an epitope on hepatocyte

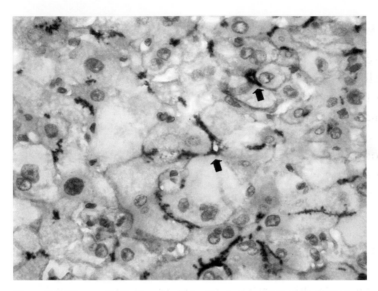

Figure 3.7 Bile canalicular immunohistochemical positivity with CD10 (*arrows*) is a feature of both benign and neoplastic liver, and can be used as evidence of hepatocellular differentiation. (CD10 immunohistochemical stain, ×400) (See color plate section.)

mitochondria. Both are highly sensitive in HCC overall, with reported sensitivity of 78–92% [8,9,10], although the more poorly differentiated and/or higher grade HCC that are diagnostically problematic are likely to be the ones that are negative [8]. Hep Par 1 and Hepatocyte are negative in nearly all CCA and metastatic adenocarcinomas. A few cases of gastric, ovarian, and lung adenocarcinomas and a few cases of neuroendocrine carcinoma/carcinoid tumors have been reported to be positive [10]. Another option is to use markers that highlight bile canaliculi, because that is a feature of hepatocellular differentiation. Two antibodies that may be used are pCEA and CD10. Biliary glycoprotein I, a protein located in bile canaliculi, cross-reacts with pCEA. Similarly, CD10, a cell surface enzyme that is normally present on the surfaces of early lymphoid cells and a few other types of normal cells, will highlight bile canaliculi, frequently with more intense staining than pCEA. Both normal and neoplastic hepatocytes may form bile canaliculi, so staining of a liver neoplasm in the characteristic bile canalicular pattern can be used as evidence of hepatocellular differentiation (Figure 3.7) [8,9,10,11,12]. Glypican-3, although not specific for liver tumors, is expressed in only a limited set of neoplasms, so it could be useful if other tumors known to be positive are not part of the differential diagnosis morphologically [5,6,7].

Fine-needle aspiration diagnosis of hepatocellular carcinoma

HCC is amenable to diagnosis by cytologic analysis of FNA specimens, as the cytologic criteria are well-described. FNA is reported to have 78.4% sensitivity and 97.4% specificity in the diagnosis of HCC [13]. Smears prepared from FNA are generally quite cellular, more so than are smears of benign liver. As bile ducts are not present in HCC, the smears lack bile ducts, unless they have been sampled from adjacent cirrhotic liver. In the latter circumstance they are not admixed with tumor cells. The same criteria apply to FNA cytologic diagnosis of HCC as to biopsy diagnosis. That is, the tumor cells must have hepatocellular differentiation and be convincingly malignant. Hepatocellular differentiation in cytologic specimens is recognized as cells that are polygonal, with dense, granular cytoplasm and well-defined cell borders. The cytoplasm may contain any of the components described earlier in text – fat droplets, Mallory's hyaline, ground-glass inclusions, or alpha-1 antitrypsin globules. Bile may be present within tumor cells or in dilated canaliculi present between tumor cells. Despite resembling hepatocytes, the nuclear features and arrangement of these cells on FNA smears differ from those of normal liver. Compared with those of non-neoplastic liver, the cells of HCC have uniformly increased ratios of nuclear-to-cytoplasmic volumes, resulting in overall cell sizes that are often smaller than normal hepatocytes. However, nuclei are larger. They characteristically have macronucleoli, sometimes larger than red blood cells. Intranuclear cytoplasmic invaginations are present in approximately half of cases, and multinucleation and mitotic figures may be present. Classically, the cells are present in trabeculae or cords from 2 to 10 cells thick, at least partially surrounded by endothelial cells (Figure 3.8). Occasionally, pseudoglandular arrangements are present, also partly surrounded by endothelial cells. Normal liver cells are generally present as small, sheetlike groups and single cells, without endothelial cells, and endothelial cells are not a feature of most other neoplasms. A second common pattern is one in which tumor nuclei are stripped of cytoplasm by the trauma of the aspiration, resulting in a smear of dissociated naked nuclei that superficially resembles a large cell lymphoma. Careful attention to the presence of a few cells that have retained their cytoplasm is important to diagnosing such cases. Poorly differentiated HCC yield cells with pleomorphic nuclei, bizarre tumor giant cells, and scant cytoplasm and without the characteristic trabecular or pseudoglandular arrangements [13,14,15]. In problematic cases, immunohistochemical study of tissue in cell block preparations can be performed in the same way as it is in needle biopsies.

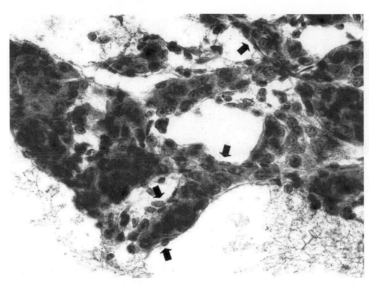

Figure 3.8 FNA of HCC yields tumor cells arranged in anastomosing cords, partially covered by endothelial cells (*arrows*). The cells have larger nuclei, less cytoplasm, and are more crowded than normal hepatocytes. (Papanicolaou stain, ×200) (See color plate section.)

Cholangiocarcinoma

CCA is a malignant neoplasm of bile duct epithelial cells. Although most CCA are of unknown etiology, strongly associated risk factors include primary sclerosing cholangitis, *Opisthorchis viverrini* infection, thorotrast exposure, choledochal cysts, and intrahepatic lithiasis [16]. In addition, chronic hepatitis C and alcoholic cirrhosis recently have been correlated with bile duct dysplasia [17]. CCA may originate outside the liver parenchyma (extrahepatic) in the right or left main bile ducts, the common bile duct, or the cystic duct. A CCA involving both the left and right hepatic ducts at their bifurcation is referred to as a Klatskin tumor or hilar CCA. Intrahepatic CCA are those that occur within the liver, with or without obvious association with a bile duct. This is the type of CCA that we will be discussing in this chapter.

Macroscopic features

Most CCA occurs in non-cirrhotic livers, and are firm, pale, usually single masses (Figure 3.9), although satellite nodules and/or multiple masses may be present. Necrosis and hemorrhage are unusual features. Foci of calcification are present in some examples. Intrahepatic spread may occur via the portal vein [18].

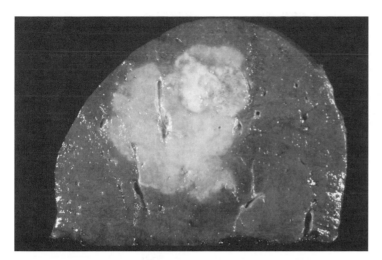

Figure 3.9 This cholangiocarcinoma is a single, non-encapsulated mass. It is dense and nearly white due to the abundant fibrous stroma that is typical of cholangiocarcinoma. (See color plate section.)

Microscopic features

Pancreaticobiliary adenocarcinomas have similar histologic features whether they are intrahepatic, extrahepatic, or pancreatic. All are composed of epithelial cells that form tubules, cell nests, trabeculae, or (less commonly) micropapillary arrangements. Tumor nests or trabeculae are separated by fibrous tissue that is characteristically abundant, especially centrally, and results in the firm, white gross appearance. Most CCA are well-differentiated, with cuboidal to columnar tumor cells. Nuclei are round to oval, with homogeneous granular chromatin. They generally lack the macronucleoli that are typical of HCC, although in some cases they are prominent. The cytoplasm may be eosinophilic or vacuolated, and intracytoplasmic or luminal mucin may be present (Figure 3.10). Bile is not formed by the tumor cells, so it should be absent unless the tumor has entrapped non-neoplastic liver parenchyma. Tumor cells infiltrate adjacent liver parenchyma by growing along sinusoids, which may result in incorporation of portal tracts by tumor stroma. CCA involving large ducts may have an intraductal papillary component, and spread along the biliary tree [18,19].

Histologic variants

Several histologic variants have been described. For the most part, these variants are not of clinical significance, as most do not imply different prognoses or

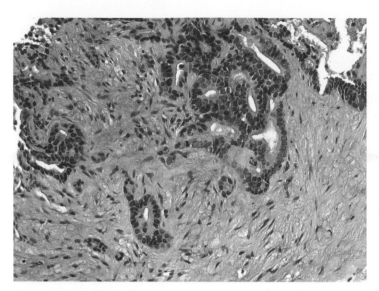

Figure 3.10 Most cholangiocarcinomas are composed of well-formed neoplastic tubules present within abundant fibrous stroma. (H&E, ×100) (See color plate section.)

management. However, the pathologist must be aware of them in order to recognize them as CCA. These variants include adenosquamous and squamous carcinomas, which have partial or diffuse squamous differentiation [18,19]. Mucinous CCA has abundant extracellular mucin, and one case has been reported to have aggressive behavior [20]. The lymphoepithelioma-like CCA, similar to lymphoepithelioma-like carcinomas of other sites, are undifferentiated carcinomas with intense lymphoplasmacytic infiltrates in the stroma and within epithelial nests. As in other sites, lymphoepithelioma-like CCA has been linked to Epstein–Barr virus and may have a slightly better prognosis [21,22]. The clear cell variant is rare, with several case reports in the English literature, and requires separation from the more common types of clear cell carcinoma, including renal cell carcinoma and clear cell HCC [23]. A sarcomatous variant is also recognized and has a significantly worse prognosis [24].

Differential diagnosis and immunohistochemistry

CCA must be distinguished from HCC and from various metastatic adenocarcinomas. Morphologic differences between CCA and HCC are usually apparent, but the distinction can be difficult in small biopsies. Hep Par 1, glypican-3, pCEA, and CD10, described earlier in this chapter, may be useful in a panel designed to make this distinction, because they should be negative or have a pattern incompatible with HCC [5,6,7,8,9,10,11,12]. CCA are generally positive with a variety of immunohistochemical markers, including cytokeratins 7, 8, 18, 19, CEA (cytoplasmic rather than canalicular), CA19–9, epithelial membrane antigen, BER-EP4, and MOC-31 [18,19,25,26]. Except for cytokeratins 8 and 18, these markers are negative in most cases of HCC, but may be positive in various metastatic adenocarcinomas from a variety of primary sites. A few antibodies with at least partial site specificity – such as thyroid transcription factor I for lung and thyroid, CDX2 for intestinal differentiation, and prostate specific antigen for prostatic origin – may be employed to investigate these possible primary sites. Cytokeratin 20 positivity combined with cytokeratin 7 negativity in an adenocarcinoma suggests a colorectal primary. Intrahepatic CCA and extrahepatic pancreaticobiliary adenocarcinomas are not only morphologically, but also immunohistochemically too similar to be separated pathologically. Unfortunately, it is often impossible to be certain of the primary site of any adenocarcinoma based on its immunohistochemical profile, and morphologic features must be considered in combination with radiographic and clinical features. Interestingly, high-molecular-weight cytokeratin K903 antibody stains 74% of CCA. Those CCA with reduced K903 expression tend to have an expansile growth pattern, medullary-type stromal reaction, and absent perineural invasion, and have better prognosis [27].

Fine-needle aspiration diagnosis of cholangiocarcinoma

Just as the histologic features of intrahepatic CCA are similar to those of extrahepatic pancreaticobiliary adenocarcinomas, the cytologic features are similar as well. Most are well-differentiated and have cells resembling normal bile duct epithelium, with columnar or honeycomb arrangements of epithelial cells, but with disorderly nuclear crowding and stratification, microacinar structures, anisonucleosis, irregular nuclear membranes, and prominent nucleoli. Less-differentiated examples may have cells with a squamoid appearance – that is, they have abundant, dense, eosinophilic cytoplasm and hyperchromatic nuclei. In general, distinction from HCC is not difficult, but exclusion of a metastatic adenocarcinoma may be difficult or impossible [28].

Combined hepatocellular and cholangiocarcinoma

Rare hepatic carcinomas (1%) have combinations of HCC and CCA [29]. These combined tumors have demographic and clinical features similar to those in patients with pure CCA, with similar rates of occurrence in viral hepatitis and chronic liver disease [30,31].

Combined HCC/CCA may resemble HCC or CCA grossly, depending on whether there is an abundant CCA component with its fibrous stroma. Unequivocal histologic evidence of both HCC and CCA must be present for the tumor to qualify for this designation, and they must be admixed; otherwise, the tumor may be synchronous HCC and CCA that are growing adjacent to each other (so-called "collision tumors"). Bile production, Hep Par I, pCEA, and CD10 staining may support the interpretation of hepatocellular differentiation, as described earlier in this chapter, and intracellular or extracellular mucin, cytokeratins 7, 19, or K903, MOC-31, or other markers of adenocarcinoma may be used to support ductular differentiation in the CCA component.

In summary, HCC and CCA comprise the most common primary malignancies of the liver. Both have associated risk factors, distinct morphologic features, and several histologic variants. A wide variety of primary tumors from other sites have a propensity to metastasize to the liver. The most common sources of metastases include pancreas, lung, and colon. Immunohistochemical stains can be helpful in suggesting the source of the metastasis, but morphology, in combination with imaging studies and clinical features, is the fundamental means of establishing a pathologic diagnosis of liver masses.

REFERENCES

1. Ishak KG, Goodman ZD, and Stocker JT. Tumors of the liver and intrahepatic bile ducts. In *Armed Forces Institute of Pathology, Atlas of Tumor Pathology*, Third Series, Fascicle 31. Washington, DC: American Registry of Pathology, 1999; **199**: 203–43.

2. Hamilton SR, and Aaltonen LA. Pathology and genetics of tumours of the digestive system. In *World Health Organization Classification of Tumours*. Lyon, France: International Agency for Research on Cancer Press, 2000; 163–66.

3. Matsuura S, Aishima S, Taguchi K, *et al.* 'Scirrhous' type hepatocellular carcinomas: A special reference to expression of cytokeratin 7 and hepatocyte paraffin 1. *Histopathology* 2005; **47**: 382–90.

4. Kurogi M, Nakashima O, Miyaaki H, Fujimoto M, and Kojiro M. Clinicopathological study of scirrhous hepatocellular carcinoma. *J Gastroenterol Hepatol* 2006; **21**: 1470–7.

5. Libbrecht L, Severi T, Cassiman D, *et al.* Glypican-3 expression distinguishes small hepatocellular carcinomas from cirrhosis, dysplastic nodules, and focal nodular hyperplasia-like nodules. *Am J Surg Pathol* 2006; **30**: 1405–11.

6. Kakar S, Gown A, Goodman ZD, and Ferrell LD. Best practices in diagnostic immunohistochemistry. Hepatocellular carcinoma versus metastatic neoplasms. *Arch Pathol Lab Med.* 2007; **131**: 1648–54.

7. Coston W, Loera S, Lau SK, *et al.* Distinction of hepatocellular carcinoma from benign hepatic mimickers using glypican-3 and CD34 immunohistochemistry. *Am J Surg Pathol* 2008; **32**: 433–44.

8. Lau SK, Prakash S, Geller SA, and Alsabeh R. Comparative immunohistochemical profile of hepatocellular carcinoma, cholangiocarcinoma, and metastatic adenocarcinoma. *Hum Pathol* 2002; **33**: 1175–81.

9. Wang L, Vuolo M, Suhrland MJ, and Schlesinger K. HepPar1, MOC-31, pCEA, mCEA, and CD10 for distinguishing hepatocellular carcinoma vs metastatic adenocarcinoma in liver fine needle aspirates. *Acta Cytol* 2006; **50**: 257–62.

10. Chu PG, Ishizawa S, Wu E, and Weiss L. Hepatocyte antigen as a marker of hepatocellular carcinoma: An immunohistochemical comparison to carcinoembryonic antigen, CD10, and alpha-fetoprotein. *Am J Surg Pathol* 2002; **26**: 978–88.

11. Morrison C, Marsh W, and Frankel WL. A comparison of CD10 to pCEA, MOC-31, and Hepatocyte for the distinction of malignant tumors in the liver. *Mod Pathol* 2002; **15**: 1279–87.

12. Wee A. Diagnostic utility of immunohistochemistry in hepatocellular carcinoma, its variants and their mimics. *Appl Immunohistochem Mol Morphol* 2006; **14**. 266–72.

13. Kuo FY, Chen WJ, Lu SN, Wang JH, and Eng HL. Fine needle aspiration cytodiagnosis of liver tumors. *Acta Cytol* 2004; **48**: 142–8.

14. DeMay RM. *The Art and Science of Cytopathology*. Chicago: ASCP Press, 1996; 1028–30.

15. de Boer WB, Segal A, Frost FA, and Sterrett GF. Cytodiagnosis of well differentiated hepatocellular carcinoma. Can indeterminate diagnoses be reduced? *Cancer Cytopathol* 1999; **87**: 270–7.

16. Shaib Y and El-Serag HB. The epidemiology of cholangiocarcinoma. *Semin Liver Dis* 2004; **24**: 115–25.

17. Torbenson M, Yeh MM, and Abraham SC. Bile duct dysplasia in the setting of chronic hepatitis C and alcohol cirrhosis. *Am J Surg Pathol* 2007; **31**: 1410–13.

18. Ishak KG, Goodman ZD, and Stocker JT. Tumors of the liver and intrahepatic bile ducts. In *Armed Forces Institute of Pathology, Atlas of Tumor Pathology*, Third Series, Fascicle 31. Washington, DC: American Registry of Pathology, 1999; 250–7.

19. Hamilton SR and Aaltonen LA. Pathology and genetics of tumours of the digestive system. In *World Health Organization Classification of Tumours*. Lyon, France: International Agency for Research on Cancer Press, 2000; 175–7.

20. Sasaki M, Nakamuma Y, Shimizu K, and Izumi R. Pathological and immunohistochemical findings in a case of mucinous cholangiocarcinoma. *Pathol Int* 1995; **45**: 781–6.

21. Jeng Y-M, Chen C-L, and Hsu H-C. Lymphoepithelioma-like cholangiocarcinoma: An Epstein-Barr virus-associated tumor. *Am J Surg Pathol* 2001; **25**: 516–20.

22. Adachi S, Morimoto O, and Kobayashi T. Case report. Lymphoepithelioma-like cholangiocarcinoma not associated with EBV. *Pathol Int* 2008; **58**: 69–74.

23. Haas S, Gutgemann I, Wolff M, and Fischer H-P. Intrahepatic clear cell cholangiocarcinoma: Immunohistochemical aspects in a very rare type of cholangiocarcinoma. *Am J Surg Pathol* 2007; **31**: 902–6.

24. Shimada M, Takenaka K, Rikimaru T, *et al.* Characteristics of sarcomatous cholangiocarcinoma of the liver. *Hepato-Gastroenterology* 2000; **47**: 956–61.

25. Sasaki A, Kawano K, Aramaki M, Nakashima K, Yoshida T, and Kitano S. Immunohistochemical expression of cytokeratins in intrahepatic cholangiocarcinoma and metastatic adenocarcinoma of the liver. *J Surg Oncol* 1999; **70**: 103–8.

26. Shimonishi T, Miyazaki K, and Nakanuma Y. Cytokeratin profile relates to histological subtypes and intrahepatic location of the intrahepatic cholangiocarcinoma and primary sites of metastatic adenocarcinoma of liver. *Histopathology* 2000; **37**: 55–63.

27. Aishima S, Asayama Y, Taguchi K, *et al.* The utility of keratin 903 as a new prognostic marker in mass-forming-type intrahepatic cholangiocarcinoma. *Mod Pathol* 2002; **15**: 1181–90.

28. DeMay RM. *The Art and Science of Cytopathology.* Chicago: ASCP Press, 1996; 1034.

29. Hamilton SR and Aaltonen LA. Pathology and genetics of tumours of the digestive system. In *World Health Organization Classification of Tumours.* Lyon, France: International Agency for Research on Cancer Press, 2000; 181.

30. Jarnagin WR, Weber S, Tickoo SK, *et al.* Combined hepatocellular and cholangiocarcinoma: Demographic, clinical, and prognostic factors. *Cancer* 2002; **94**(7): 2040–6.

31. Portolani N, Baiocchi GL, Goniglio A, *et al.* Intrahepatic cholangiocarcinoma and combined hepatocellular-cholangiocarcinoma: A Western experience. *Ann Surg Oncol* 2008; **15**: 1880–90.

4

Radiological diagnosis of hepatocellular carcinoma

Jonathon M. Willatt, Hero K. Hussain, and Isaac R. Francis

Contrast-enhanced computed tomography (CT) and magnetic resonance imaging (MRI) perform the major roles in the diagnosis of hepatocellular carcinoma (HCC) alongside alpha-fetoprotein (AFP) serology and biopsy. There is also increasing use of contrast-enhanced ultrasound (CEUS) for the diagnosis of HCC. Accessibility to each modality and expertise determine which is used as the major imaging tool for the diagnosis of HCC. In the context of the rapid increase in the incidence of HCC, it is important to recognize that there will be increasing reliance on imaging tools to diagnose and stage tumors.

Two sets of clinical practice guidelines published in the western literature form the basis of radiologic diagnosis of HCC in both Europe and the United States. These are the European Association for the Study of the Liver (EASL) guidelines formed at the single-topic conference on HCC in 2000 [1] and the American Association for the Study of Liver Diseases (AASLD) practice guideline published in 2005 [2].

Ultrasound

The role of ultrasound is primarily in the surveillance of at-risk patients [3]. The introduction of contrast agents has presented new opportunities for ultrasound specialists in the diagnosis of HCC [4]. HCC shows strong intratumoral enhancement in the arterial phase followed by rapid washout with an isoechoic or hypoechoic appearance in the portal and delayed phases (Figure 4.1). Regenerative and dysplastic nodules do not show early contrast enhancement. Selective arterial enhancement has been shown in 91–96% of lesions confirming a high sensitivity in identifying the arterial neoangiogenesis of HCC [5,6,7,8]. Contrast agents are limited, however, in assessing the whole of the liver because only one lesion can be assessed after a single injection. They are also not yet approved by the U.S. Food & Drug Administration (FDA) for clinical use for this indication.

Primary Carcinomas of the Liver, ed. Hero K. Hussain and Isaac R. Francis. Published by Cambridge University Press. © Cambridge University Press 2010.

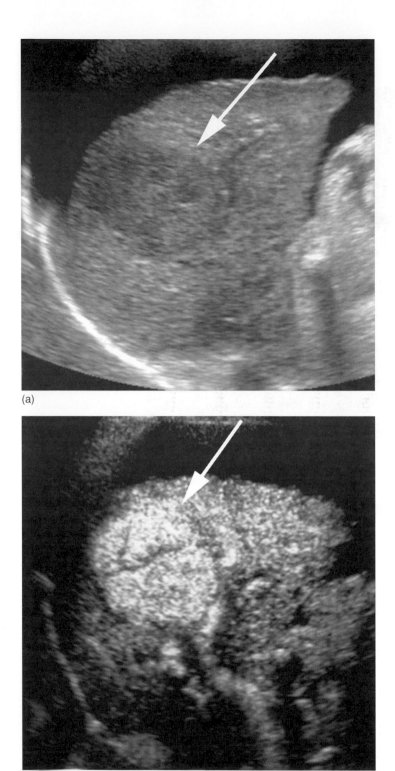

(a)

(b)

Figure 4.1 (a–c): Unenhanced ultrasound image (a) demonstrates a 3.5 cm-HCC (*arrow*) in the right hepatic lobe. Following the administration of contrast there is arterial uptake (b) and delayed washout (c). Courtesy of Dr. Tae Kyoung Kim, Department of Medical Imaging, University of Toronto.

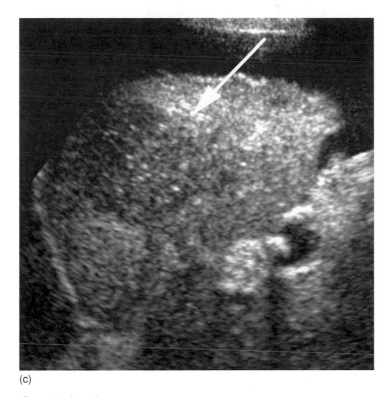

(c)

Figure 4.1 (*cont.*)

Computed tomography and magnetic resonance imaging

There is variability in the accuracy of both CT and MRI with regard to the size of HCC detected, but there is greater confidence in the diagnosis of larger lesions for both modalities [9,10].

The process of neoangiogenesis or arterial recruitment dictates the main imaging feature of HCC, which is arterial enhancement [11]. Arterial enhancement is considered an essential characteristic of HCC and is used as the only radiological feature for the non-invasive diagnosis of HCC by the United Network for Organ Sharing, the organization responsible for transplant liver allocation in the United States [12]. Arterial enhancement tends to be heterogeneous in large lesions and homogeneous in small lesions [13], and is related to the development of arterial supply to the tumor by non-triadal arteries.

HCC will characteristically appear hypointense or hypodense during the delayed phase following intravenous contrast administration due to the diminution in the portal tracts and replacement by non-triadal arteries [13]. This feature is particularly

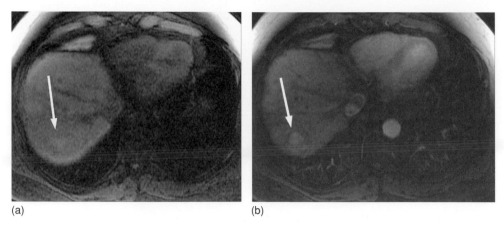

(a)   (b)

Figure 4.2 (a and b): A 1.7 cm HCC (*arrows*) in the right hepatic lobe, segment VII, demonstrates high SI on precontrast fat-saturated T1W three-dimensional gradient-recalled echo (3-D GRE) image (a) and hypervascularity in the arterial phase of enhancement (b).

useful because there are several other entities that are not HCC but can demonstrate arterial enhancement. A small proportion of dysplastic nodules receive their supply from the hepatic artery, and the delayed phase can therefore play an important role in distinguishing these precancerous nodules from HCC. At times, however, both histologically and radiologically it can be difficult to differentiate some dysplastic nodules from small HCC.

Radiological MRI criteria favoring malignancy in a nodule are a size larger than 3 cm, hyperintensity on T2-weighted (T2W) imaging, delayed hypointensity or low attenuation "washout," a delayed enhancing rim on postcontrast imaging, and rapid interval growth [14].

HCC has variable signal intensity (SI) on unenhanced T1-weighted (T1W) and T2W MRI [15,16]. High SI on T1W imaging (Figure 4.2) is attributed to intratumoral fat, hemorrhage, copper, glycogen, or zinc in the surrounding parenchyma [15,17]. Fat content leads to signal loss on opposed phase imaging [18]. Moderate high SI on T2W imaging is quite specific for HCC as dysplastic nodules are not hyperintense unless they have undergone infarction [14,15,19]. However, HCC can be difficult to detect on T2W imaging because of tumor isointensity to liver parenchyma and heterogeneity of the cirrhotic liver, which obscures tumors when they are mildly hyperintense or isointense in signal relative to adjacent parenchyma [20,21].

Other lesions that exhibit arterial enhancement can mimic HCC – for example, areas of transient hepatic attenuation (intensity) difference caused by

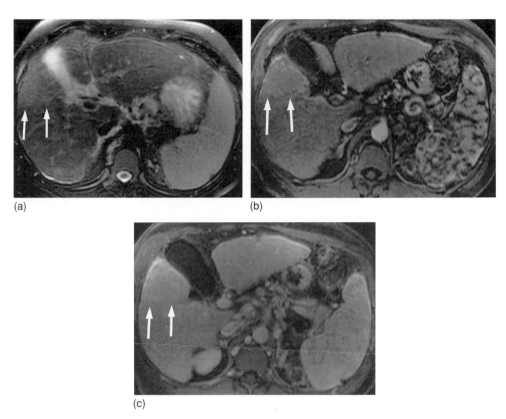

Figure 4.3 (a–c): Wedge-shaped area adjacent to the gallbladder (*arrows*) demonstrates high SI relative to liver parenchyma on T2W fast spin-echo (FSE) imaging (a), hypervascularity in the arterial phase following gadolinium administration (b), and retention of contrast in the delayed phase (c) on fat-suppressed T1W 3-D GRE images, consistent with confluent hepatic fibrosis.

non-tumorous arterioportal shunts [22,23] or by focal obstruction of a distal parenchymal portal vein as often seen in the cirrhotic liver. Focal confluent hepatic fibrosis (Figure 4.3) can create a masslike lesion that can be mistaken for HCC, especially in cirrhosis secondary to primary sclerosing cholangitis [24], but can be distinguished by its subcapsular location, wedge-shaped morphology, delayed enhancement, and associated capsular retraction. Atypical hemangiomas [25], focal nodular hyperplasia-like lesions, and hepatic adenoma, although less commonly seen in the cirrhotic liver than in the normal liver, can also create diagnostic uncertainty.

Accurate radiological diagnosis of HCC is important because decisions regarding curative therapy (including radiofrequency ablation, surgical resection, or transplantation) are made based on the imaging findings. Lesions detected in high-risk populations (cirrhotics and chronic hepatitis B carriers) on surveillance

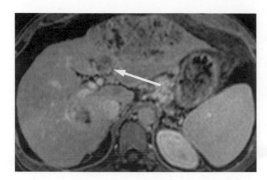

Figure 4.4 Delayed phase, fat-suppressed T1W 3-D GRE gadolinium-enhanced MRI shows delayed hypointensity "washout" in a large HCC occupying the lateral segment of the left hepatic lobe. There is expansile tumor thrombus in the left portal vein (*arrow*).

ultrasound require further evaluation with contrast-enhanced studies (MRI, CT, or ultrasound).

Diagnosis of hepatocellular carcinoma in arterially hypervascular lesions according to size

Lesions greater than or equal to 2 cm in diameter

An arterially enhancing mass measuring greater than or equal to 2 cm and demonstrating venous or delayed hypointensity "washout" in a cirrhotic liver is highly likely to be HCC, and biopsy is not essential [9,10].

Very large HCC is characterized by a more variable pattern – the so-called "mosaic pattern." A mosaic pattern is created by confluent nodules separated by fibrous septa and areas of necrosis. Generally, larger HCC tend to be of higher SI, are less arterially hypervascular, and show more pronounced washout compared to smaller tumors [26,27].

Diffuse type HCC constitutes up to 13% of cases of HCC [28] and appears as an extensive, heterogeneous, permeative hepatic tumor often associated with portal venous thrombosis (Figure 4.4). These tumors have a patchy or nodular early enhancement pattern and can be difficult to detect on contrast-enhanced CT (Figure 4.5) and on T1W or T2W imaging because of their similar signal and degree of enhancement to the underlying nodular pattern of the liver. These tumors tend to be most conspicuous in the late phases of enhancement due to prominent washout [28].

In the setting of cirrhosis, both contrast-enhanced CT and MRI are highly accurate in the diagnosis of HCC measuring 2 cm or larger [29,30]. The positive predictive value of the combined clinical (AFP) and radiological findings exceeds 95% [1]. For the radiological diagnosis of HCC in cirrhosis, the EASL guidelines published

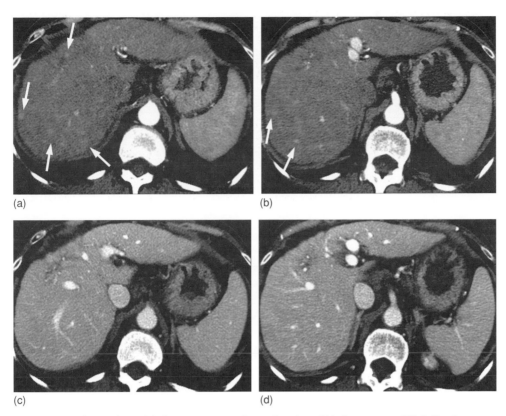

(a)   (b)

(c)   (d)

Figure 4.5 (a–d): Axial arterial phase contrast enhanced CT (a and b) shows several ill-defined arterially enhancing lesions in a liver that shows morphologic features of cirrhosis. AFP was 1540. However, there was no delayed hypointensity on the later phases (c and d). Subsequent angiography and lipiodol CT (not shown) demonstrated diffuse HCC in the right lobe.

in 2001 recommend confirmation of the presence of the mass and arterial hyper-vascularity on two imaging modalities (ultrasound, CT, MRI, or angiography) or on a single modality if the AFP is greater than 400 ng/mL [1].

The more recent AASLD guidelines published in 2005 [2] further refine the EASL guidelines and require only one contrast-enhanced imaging modality (CT, MRI, or ultrasound) for the radiological diagnosis of HCC greater than or equal to 2 cm in the setting of cirrhosis if the mass shows typical features of malignancy including arterial hypervascularity and venous washout [hypodensity/hypointensity relative to adjacent liver parenchyma in the venous and/or delayed phase of enhancement (Figure 4.6)], or if the AFP is more than 200 ng/ml [11,14,31]. The recommendations state that such examinations should be conducted using state-of-the-art equipment and read by radiologists with extensive expertise in liver radiology.

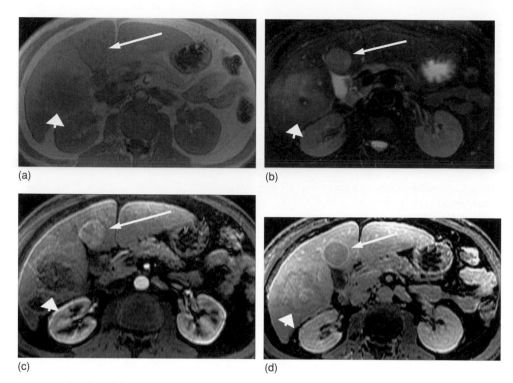

Figure 4.6 (a–d): Axial T1W GRE in-phase (a), T2W FSE (b), and arterial (c) and venous (d) phase gadolinium-enhanced, fat-suppressed T1W 3-D GRE images show two lesions. The 3.5 cm lesion in the medial segment of the left lobe (*arrow*) was an HCC. Relative to liver parenchyma, this lesion is low in SI on T1W imaging, high in SI on T2W imaging, enhances in the arterial phases, becomes hypointense on delayed postgadolinium imaging, and has a delayed enhancing rim. These features are typical for HCC. By contrast, the 8 cm lesion (*arrowhead*) in the right lobe demonstrates a thin irregular rim of enhancement and central hypointensity on the arterial phase, and delayed filling of the central components. This was a cholangiocarcinoma.

Biopsy is recommended for lesions larger than 2 cm if the vascular profile on dynamic imaging is not characteristic or if a suspicious nodule is detected in a non-cirrhotic liver.

The presence of a delayed enhancing rim and hyperintensity on T2W MRI increases the specificity of the diagnosis [14]. The guidelines also state that other radiological tests, such as lipiodol angiography, that have been used to diagnose HCC are of less value for small HCC, and that standard angiography and CT arterioportal angiography (CTAP) should not be routinely performed.

Tumor growth beyond 2 to 3 cm is usually associated with microscopic vascular invasion or satellite lesions, which are predictors of recurrence after initial therapy [32].

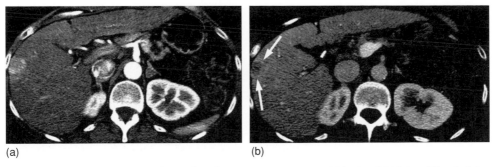

(a)   (b)

Figure 4.7 (a and b): Contrast-enhanced CT demonstrates a 1.9 cm HCC in the right lobe with arterial enhancement (a) and delayed hypointensity (b). There is a thin enhancing rim on the delayed phase (*arrows*). Note a left adrenal nodule.

Lesions 1 to less than 2 cm in diameter

Small HCC measuring 1 to less than 2 cm in the cirrhotic liver is more difficult to diagnose because such lesions do not always display the typical imaging features of a tumor (arterial hypervascularity and delayed washout), and small, benign, arterially enhancing lesions are prevalent in cirrhosis. However, detection of these tumors is the goal of surveillance programs that assess patients every 6 to 12 months. Small tumors are less likely to have microscopic vascular or local parenchymal spread; therefore, they respond favorably to local therapies (ablation and resection), which improve outcome [33].

Arterially enhancing nodules measuring 1 to less than 2 cm found in the cirrhotic liver have a high probability of being HCC if they demonstrate the typical imaging characteristics, including arterial enhancement, venous or delayed hypointensity or hypodensity washout (Figure 4.7), delayed enhancing rim, and hyperintense signal on T2W imaging. However, small HCC (≤ 1.5 cm) are frequently isoattenuating on unenhanced CT, and isointense on T1W and T2W MRI. Moreover, many do not show delayed washout and are therefore only detected in the arterial phase [16]. The imaging characteristics of those lesions that demonstrate arterial enhancement without delayed hypointensity or low attenuation overlap with those of high-grade dysplastic nodules and with those of other benign nodules. Studies have shown that many of these lesions will remain stable or may regress over time, indicating that they are not HCC [34,35,36,37].

Sometimes, tumors also lack arterial hypervascularity (isovascular or hypovascular tumors) (Figure 4.8). This probably reflects the stage of carcinogenesis within the nodule where there has been partial or complete loss of the normal portal tract with

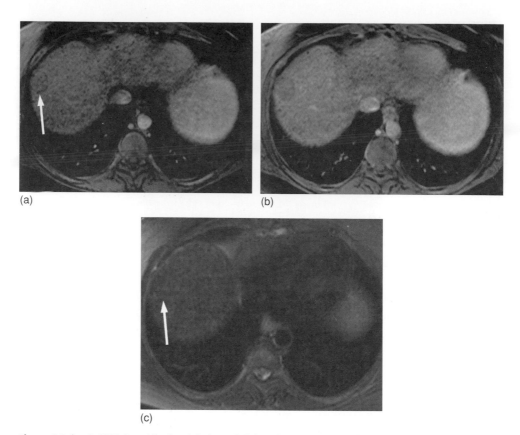

(a)   (b)

(c)

Figure 4.8 (a–c): HCC (2 cm) in the right hepatic lobe of intermediate SI to liver on the T1W 3-D GRE gadolinium-enhanced arterial phase image (a) and low SI on the delayed phase image (b) (*arrows*). This lesion was also isointense to liver parenchyma on T2W imaging (c). This is an isovascular HCC.

no associated increased arterialization to cause hyperintensity in the arterial phase [38,39]. Suspicion therefore rests on delayed hypointensity or hypoattenuation, or interval enlargement of the nodule.

The EASL guidelines recommend that biopsies should be taken of these suspicious nodules (1 to <2 cm) [1]. However, image-guided biopsy becomes less useful as lesions get smaller as these lesions are more difficult to target and may be missed by the biopsy needle. In addition, pathology results may be equivocal [40]. A positive result is therefore useful for management decisions, but a negative result cannot be taken as conclusive. The AASLD guidelines suggest that nodules between 1 and 2 cm found on ultrasound screening of a cirrhotic liver should be investigated further with two dynamic contrast-enhanced studies – CT, MRI, or ultrasound [2,37]. If the appearances are typical of HCC (i.e., hypervascular with washout)

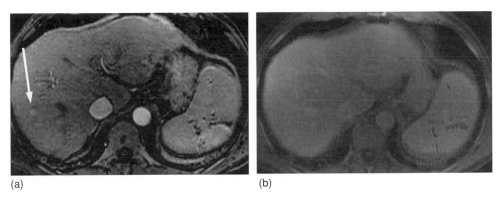

(a)   (b)

Figure 4.9 (a and b): T1W, fat-suppressed 3-D GRE gadolinium-enhanced arterial phase image (a) demonstrates an 8 mm arterial enhancing lesion (*arrow*). There is no concomitant hypointensity on the delayed phase (b). This was not present on follow-up examinations.

on both modalities, the lesion should be treated as HCC. If the vascular profile is not concordant among techniques or the imaging findings are not characteristic, a biopsy should be taken of the lesion. Patients with a negative biopsy should continue with surveillance at three-month intervals or have a repeat biopsy.

Lesions less than 1 cm

Arterially enhancing lesions measuring less than 1 cm in the cirrhotic liver are even less likely to be HCC. Those without corroborative features, such as delayed hypointensity/hypodensity and a delayed enhancing rim, are unlikely to be HCC [41,42]. Taking a biopsy of these lesions is extremely difficult, and a negative result is of little value. These lesions should be followed, usually at a 6-month interval, for up to 2 years to demonstrate resolution (Figure 4.9), lack of interval growth, or change in imaging features [2]. If they do not show growth over a period of 2 years they are unlikely to represent HCC. Many of these small nodules disappear on follow-up scans, indicating that they are transient phenomena such as vascular perfusion defects.

Diagnostic accuracy

Two explant studies, both published since 2001, compare the accuracies of ultrasound, CT, and MRI for the detection of HCC and show that contrast-enhanced MRI is the most sensitive technique for detecting liver nodules. Rode *et al.* [43] prospectively assessed the sensitivities for nodules measuring 8 to 35 mm in patients awaiting transplantation, and found that MRI had higher sensitivity (77%) than CT (54%) or ultrasound (54%). The specificity of MRI was lower at 57% compared with 93% for CT and 95% for ultrasound. Libbrecht *et al.* [44] found MRI to have higher sensitivity (70%) than CT (50%) or ultrasound (40%). The specificity of MRI (82%) was comparable to that of CT (79%) and lower than that of ultrasound (100%). In this study, HCC sizes ranged from 2 to 40 mm, and one liver contained up to 30 HCC. The conclusions of both of these studies were that currently used imaging techniques cannot accurately determine the exact tumor burden in cirrhotic patients, that lesions smaller than 1 cm are usually not seen on ultrasound, and that lesions smaller than 5 mm are usually not shown on CT or MRI. Because of these shortcomings, patients still undergo transplantation even though they exceed the tumor number limit (up to three tumors each smaller than 3 cm), and others are still explanted despite having no malignant lesion.

Colli *et al.* [45] performed a systematic review of 9 MRI studies, 10 CT studies, and 14 ultrasound studies, as well as AFP studies, and found that although ultrasound is highly specific for HCC detection, it is insufficiently sensitive to support an effective surveillance program. MRI was found to be the most sensitive of the three tests. This study gives no indication as to the variation in accuracy dependent on the size of the HCC.

Most studies that aim to evaluate the diagnostic accuracy of a technique are limited because they include only patients with known HCC, thereby introducing bias. However, a prospective investigation conducted between 2003 and 2006 assessed the diagnostic accuracy of both CEUS and contrast-enhanced MRI for small solitary nodules measuring 5 to 20 mm using the non-invasive criteria proposed by the AASLD in 89 patients with pathologic correlation [37]. The diagnostic accuracy of MRI alone (sensitivity 62–85%, specificity 90–97%) was slightly greater than that of CEUS (sensitivity 52–78%, specificity 86–93%) for conclusively malignant lesions (those possessing arterial enhancement and venous washout) and for suspicious lesions (those possessing arterial enhancement only). However, the combined sensitivity and specificity of CEUS and MRI together was 33% and 100%, respectively, for conclusive and suspicious lesions. This study shows that, for a lesion of 2 cm or less, a single test can result in the wrong diagnosis and that the use of two diagnostic techniques eliminated false positives. However, the sensitivity of both techniques used together is low, thus, many lesions remain dependent on biopsy for confirmation. This low figure is accounted for by the fact that many small HCC do not demonstrate delayed washout. Unfortunately, performing two diagnostic studies may not be feasible in many patients. Techniques such as lipiodol CT or angiography have a limited role in the diagnosis of HCC [46].

New magnetic resonance imaging techniques

The results of new MRI techniques using liver-specific contrast agents without or with gadolinium are promising [47,48,49,50]. These agents exploit the cellular properties of HCC and comprise two groups: the superparamagnetic iron oxide (SPIO) agents, which are targeted to the reticuloendothelial system, and the hepatocyte-specific agents, which are taken up by hepatocytes and excreted in bile. The degree of biliary excretion varies among these agents and is highest with gadoxetate disodium. Some of these hepatocyte-specific agents (gadobenate dimeglumine and gadoxetate disodium) have vascular properties as well and can be used as extracellular gadolinium agents. Both of these agents offer the advantage of higher T1 relaxivity (i.e., brighter) compared with extracellular gadolinium agents when used at the same dose. This property may help to increase the conspicuity of hypervascular lesions, or it can be used to reduce the dose of contrast while maintaining the same effect as the extracellular agents.

Uptake of SPIO contrast manifests as signal loss on T2W and T2*W images due to the T2 shortening effect of the agent. Uptake of hepatocyte-specific agents by functioning hepatocytes manifests as an increase in the SI of the liver parenchyma leading to increased conspicuity of HCC, which typically does not show contrast uptake in the hepatobiliary phase images acquired 20 minutes to 3 hours after intravenous administration of contrast using a three-dimensional T1W gradient–echo sequence. Most HCCs, except for the well-differentiated tumors, do not have functioning Kupffer cells or hepatocytes and do not take up either contrast agent. With hepatocyte-specific agents, a classic HCC (Figure 4.10) will be hypervascular in the arterial phase, as with other extracellular agents, and hypointense relative to liver parenchyma in the delayed hepatobiliary phase. False-negative results can be seen in well-differentiated HCC, which can contain functioning Kupffer cells and hepatocytes and enhance with both agents.

Recent studies [47,48] using two contrast techniques (SPIO and gadolinium) have shown high sensitivity (81–94%) and positive predictive value (PPV) (81–100%) for HCC. The double-contrast technique involves the sequential administration of SPIO and gadolinium, thereby providing information on the vascularity and the Kupffer cell density on the same image. In the study by Kim *et al.* [48], these results were similar to those achieved with CT hepatic arteriography and CTAP. In a recent review of all techniques [49], the double-contrast technique was shown to have higher overall sensitivity for the detection of HCC compared to spiral CT, gadolinium-enhanced MRI, and SPIO only enhanced MRI. Of note, the only FDA approved SPIO contrast agent, ferumoxides (Feridex), has been discontinued

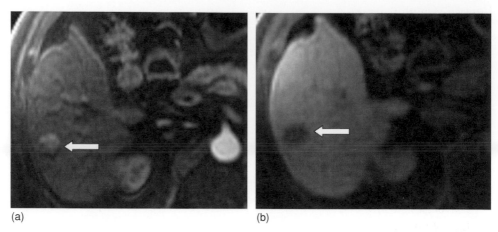

(a)   (b)

Figure 4.10 (a and b): A 1.2 cm HCC in the posterior right lobe (*arrow*) on T1W 3-D GRE images. The tumor shows intense enhancement in the arterial phase (a) following the injection of the hepatocyte-specific agent gadoxetate disodium, due to the vascular property of the agent. There is no contrast uptake by the tumor in the hepatobiliary phase of enhancement 20 minutes after contrast administration (b) due to the lack of normal functioning hepatocytes and bile ducts.

in the United States. Early results with the new hepatocyte-specific agents [50] are promising, but more studies are needed to validate these early observations. Data on the role of diffusion-weighted imaging for the detection of HCC are still preliminary [51,52].

Summary

The EASL 2000 Conference proposed a set of criteria to establish HCC diagnosis in patients with cirrhosis. These criteria were based on the observation of a hypervascular profile of the nodule by two dynamic imaging techniques that included CT, MRI, and CEUS. However, these non-invasive criteria were restricted to tumors larger than 2 cm. Below this cutoff, biopsy was mandatory to establish a diagnosis of HCC.

The recognition of the role of contrast washout or delayed hypointensity/hypoattenuation led to the refinement of these criteria in the AASLD guidelines and in the unpublished consensus of the EASL experts who met in 2005 [33]. According to these criteria, for a nodule greater than 2 cm in size, which demonstrates arterial enhancement and washout in the venous phase, a single imaging technique is enough to establish the diagnosis of HCC whereas for nodules between 1 and 2 cm, correlative findings on two contrast-enhanced imaging techniques still should be required. If these criteria are not met, biopsy remains necessary. If biopsy is unfeasible or its results are negative, serial follow-up imaging to assess for interval growth is necessary. Disappearance or stability of the lesion for at least 2 years indicates benignity.

There are promising early results using new liver specific and combination contrast agents for the detection of HCC on MRI. More studies are needed to confirm these early observations.

REFERENCES

1. Bruix J, Sherman M, Llovet JM, *et al.* Clinical management of hepatocellular carcinoma. Conclusions of the Barcelona-2000 EASL conference. European Association for the Study of the Liver. *J Hepatol* 2001; **35**(3): 421–30.

2. Bruix J and Sherman M. Management of hepatocellular carcinoma. *Hepatology* 2005; **42**(5): 1208–36.

3. Zhang BH, Yang BH, and Tang ZY. Randomized controlled trial of screening for hepatocellular carcinoma. *J Cancer Res Clin Oncol* 2004; **130**(7): 417–22.

4. Fracanzani AL, Burdick L, Borzio M, *et al.* Contrast-enhanced Doppler ultrasonography in the diagnosis of hepatocellular carcinoma and premalignant lesions in patients with cirrhosis. *Hepatology* 2001; **34**(6): 1109–12.

5. Albrecht T, Blomley M, Bolondi L, *et al.* Guidelines for the use of contrast agents in ultrasound. *Ultraschall Med* 2004; **25**(4): 249–56.

6. Nicolau C, Vilana R, and Bru C. The use of contrast-enhanced ultrasound in the management of the cirrhotic patient and for detection of HCC. *Eur Radiol* 2004; **14**(Suppl 8): P63–71.

7. Gaiani S, Celli N, Piscaglia F, *et al.* Usefulness of contrast-enhanced perfusional sonography in the assessment of hepatocellular carcinoma hypervascular at spiral computed tomography. *J Hepatol* 2004; **41**(3): 421–6.

8. Quaia E, Calliada F, Bertolotto M, *et al.* Characterization of focal liver lesions with contrast-specific US modes and a sulfur hexafluoride-filled microbubble contrast agent: Diagnostic performance and confidence. *Radiology* 2004; **232**(2): 420–30.

9. Levy I, Greig PD, Gallinger S, Langer B, and Sherman M. Resection of hepatocellular carcinoma without preoperative tumor biopsy. *Ann Surg* 2001; **234**(2): 206–9.

10. Torzilli G, Minagawa M, Takayama T, *et al.* Accurate preoperative evaluation of liver mass lesions without fine-needle biopsy. *Hepatology* 1999; **30**(4): 889–93.

11. Marrero JA, Hussain HK, Nghiem HV, Umar R, Fontana RJ, and Lok AS. Improving the prediction of hepatocellular carcinoma in cirrhotic patients with an arterially-enhancing liver mass. *Liver Transpl* 2005; **11**(3): 281–9.

12. Sharing UNfO. The Organ Placement Process: Resources and policies – policy 3.6. 2005 [cited July 30, 2006]. Available from: http://www.unos.org/policiesandbylaws/policies.asp?resources=true

13. Yamashita Y, Mitsuzaki K, Yi T, *et al.* Small hepatocellular carcinoma in patients with chronic liver damage: Prospective comparison of detection with dynamic MR imaging and helical CT of the whole liver. *Radiology* 1996; **200**(1): 79–84.

14. Krinsky GA and Lee VS. MR imaging of cirrhotic nodules. *Abdom Imaging* 2000; **25**(5): 471–82.

15. Earls JP, Theise ND, Weinreb JC, *et al.* Dysplastic nodules and hepatocellular carcinoma: Thin-section MR imaging of explanted cirrhotic livers with pathologic correlation. *Radiology* 1996; **201**(1): 207–14.

16. Kelekis NL, Semelka RC, Worawattanakul S, *et al.* Hepatocellular carcinoma in North America: A multiinstitutional study of appearance on T1-weighted, T2-weighted, and serial gadolinium-enhanced gradient-echo images. *AJR Am J Roentgenol* 1998; **170**(4): 1005–13.

17. Kelekis NL, Semelka RC, and Woosley JT. Malignant lesions of the liver with high signal intensity on T1-weighted MR images. *J Magn Reson Imaging* 1996; **6**(2): 291–4.

18. Mitchell DG, Palazzo J, Hann HW, Rifkin MD, Burk DL, Jr., and Rubin R. Hepatocellular tumors with high signal on T1-weighted MR images: Chemical shift MR imaging and histologic correlation. *J Comput Assist Tomogr* 1991; **15**(5): 762–9.

19. Kim T, Baron RL, and Nalesnik MA. Infarcted regenerative nodules in cirrhosis: CT and MR imaging findings with pathologic correlation. *AJR Am J Roentgenol* 2000; **175**(4): 1121–5.

20. Hussain HK, Syed I, Nghiem HV, *et al.* T2-weighted MR imaging in the assessment of cirrhotic liver. *Radiology* 2004; **230**(3): 637–44.

21. Efremidis SC, Hytiroglou P, and Matsui O. Enhancement patterns and signal-intensity characteristics of small hepatocellular carcinoma in cirrhosis: Pathologic basis and diagnostic challenges. *Eur Radiol* 2007; **17**: 2969–82.

22. Yu JS, Kim KW, Sung KB, Lee JT, and Yoo HS. Small arterial-portal venous shunts: A cause of pseudolesions at hepatic imaging. *Radiology* 1997; **203**(3): 737–42.

23. Yu JS, Lee JH, Chung JJ, Kim JH, and Kim KW. Small hypervascular hepatocellular carcinoma: Limited value of portal and delayed phases on dynamic magnetic resonance imaging. *Acta Radiol* 2008; **16**: 1–9.

24. Dodd GD, 3rd, Baron RL, Oliver JH, 3rd, and Federle MP. Spectrum of imaging findings of the liver in end-stage cirrhosis: Part II, focal abnormalities. *AJR Am J Roentgenol* 1999; **173**(5): 1185–92.

25. Brancatelli G, Federle MP, Blachar A, and Grazioli L. Hemangioma in the cirrhotic liver: Diagnosis and natural history. *Radiology* 2001; **219**(1): 69–74.

26. Ito K. Hepatocellular carcinoma: Conventional MRI findings including gadolinium-enhanced dynamic imaging. *Eur J Radiol* 2006; **58**(2): 186–99.

27. Van Den Bos IC, Hussain SM, Dwarkasing RS, *et al.* MR imaging of hepatocellular carcinoma: Relationship between lesion size and imaging findings, including signal intensity and dynamic enhancement patterns. *J Magn Reson Imaging* 2007; **26**: 1548–55.

28. Kanematsu M, Semelka RC, Leonardou P, Mastropasqua M, and Lee JK. Hepatocellular carcinoma of diffuse type: MR imaging findings and clinical manifestations. *J Magn Reson Imaging* 2003; **18**(2): 189–95.

29. Krinsky GA, Lee VS, Theise ND, *et al.* Hepatocellular carcinoma and dysplastic nodules in patients with cirrhosis: Prospective diagnosis with MR imaging and explantation correlation. *Radiology* 2001; **219**(2): 445–54.

30. Taouli B, Losada M, Holland A, and Krinsky G. Magnetic resonance imaging of hepatocellular carcinoma. *Gastroenterology* 2004; **127**(5 Suppl 1): S144–52.

31. Freeny PC, Grossholz M, Kaakaji K, and Schmiedl UP. Significance of hyperattenuating and contrast-enhancing hepatic nodules detected in the cirrhotic liver during arterial phase helical CT in pre-liver transplant patients: Radiologic-histopathologic correlation of explanted livers. *Abdom Imaging* 2003; **28**(3): 333–46.

32. Llovet JM, Burroughs A, and Bruix J. Hepatocellular carcinoma. *Lancet* 2003; **362**(9399): 1907–17.

33. Arii S, Yamaoka Y, Futagawa S, *et al.* Results of surgical and nonsurgical treatment for small-sized hepatocellular carcinomas: A retrospective and nationwide survey in Japan. The Liver Cancer Study Group of Japan. *Hepatology* 2000; **32**: 1224–9.

34. Martin J, Puig J, Darnell A, and Donoso L. Magnetic resonance of focal liver lesions in hepatic cirrhosis and chronic hepatitis. *Semin Ultrasound CT MR.* 2002; **23**(1): 62–78.

35. Mueller GC, Hussain HK, Carlos RC, Nghiem HV, and Francis IR. Effectiveness of MR imaging in characterizing small hepatic lesions: Routine versus expert interpretation. *AJR Am J Roentgenol* 2003; **180**(3): 673–80.

36. Shimizu A, Ito K, Koike S, Fujita T, Shimizu K, and Matsunaga N. Cirrhosis or chronic hepatitis: Evaluation of small (< or = 2-cm) early-enhancing hepatic lesions with serial contrast-enhanced dynamic MR imaging. *Radiology* 2003; **226**(2): 550–5.

37. Forner A, Vilana R, Ayuso C, *et al.* Diagnosis of hepatic nodules 20 mm or smaller in cirrhosis: Prospective validation of the noninvasive diagnostic criteria for hepatocellular carcinoma. *Hepatology* 2008; **47**(1): 97–104.

38. Bolondi L, Gaiani S, Celli N, *et al.* Characterization of small nodules in cirrhosis by assessment of vascularity: The problem of hypovascular hepatocellular carcinoma. *Hepatology* 2005; **42**(1): 27–34.

39. Matsui O. Imaging of multistep human hepatocarcinogenesis by CT during intra-arterial contrast injection. *Intervirology* 2004; **47**(3–5): 271–6.

40. Kojiro M. Focus on dysplastic nodules and early hepatocellular carcinoma: An Eastern point of view. *Liver Transpl* 2004; **10**(2 Suppl 1): S3–8.

41. Byrnes V, Shi H, Kiryu S, Rofsky NM, and Afdhal NH. The clinical outcome of small (<20 mm) arterially enhancing nodules on MRI in the cirrhotic liver. *Am J Gastroenterol* 2007; **102**(8): 1654–9.

42. Jeong YY, Mitchell DG, and Kamishima T. Small (<20 mm) enhancing hepatic nodules seen on arterial phase MR imaging of the cirrhotic liver: Clinical implications. *AJR Am J Roentgenol* 2002; **178**(6): 1327–34.

43. Rode A, Bancel B, Douek P, *et al.* Small nodule detection in cirrhotic livers: Evaluation with US, spiral CT, and MRI and correlation with pathologic examination of explanted liver. *J Comput Assist Tomogr* 2001; **25**(3): 327–36.

44. Libbrecht L, Bielen D, Verslype C, *et al.* Focal lesions in cirrhotic explant livers: Pathological evaluation and accuracy of pretransplantation imaging examinations. *Liver Transpl* 2002; **8**(9): 749–61.

45. Colli A, Fraquelli M, Casazza G, *et al.* Accuracy of ultrasonography, spiral CT, magnetic resonance, and alpha-fetoprotein in diagnosing hepatocellular carcinoma: A systematic review. *Am J Gastroenterol* 2006; **101**(3): 513–23.

46. Bizollon T, Rode A, Bancel B, *et al.* Diagnostic value and tolerance of lipiodol-computed tomography for the detection of small hepatocellular carcinoma: Correlation with pathologic examination of explanted livers. *J Hepatol* 1998; **28**(3): 491–6.

47. Hanna RF, Kased N, Kwan SW, *et al.* Double-contrast MRI for accurate staging of hepatocellular carcinoma in patients with cirrhosis. *AJR Am J Roentgenol* 2008; **190**: 47–57.

48. Kim YK, Kwak HS, Han YM, and Kim CS. Usefulness of combining sequentially acquired gadobenate dimeglumine-enhanced magnetic resonance imaging and resovist-enhanced magnetic resonance imaging for the detection of hepatocellular carcinoma: Comparison with computed tomography hepatic arteriography and computed tomography arterioportography using 16-slice multidetector computed tomography. *J Comput Assist Tomogr* 2007; **31**: 702–11.

49. Kim SH, Choi BI, Lee JY, *et al.* Diagnostic accuracy of multi-/single-detector row CT and contrast-enhanced MRI in the detection of hepatocellular carcinomas meeting the Milan criteria before liver transplantation. *Intervirology* 2008; **51**(Suppl 1): 52–60.

50. Choi SH, Lee JM, Yu NC, *et al.* Hepatocellular carcinoma in liver transplantation candidates: Detection with gadobenate dimeglumine-enhanced MRI. *AJR Am J Roentgenol* 2008; **191**: 529–36.

51. Bruegel M, Holzapfel K, Gaa J, *et al.* Characterization of focal liver lesions by ADC measurements using a respiratory triggered diffusion-weighted single-shot echo-planar MR imaging technique. *Eur J Radiol* 2008; **18**: 477–85.

52. Parikh T, Drew SJ, Lee VS, *et al.* Focal liver lesion detection and characterization with diffusion-weighted MR imaging: Comparison with standard breath-hold T2-weighted imaging. *Radiology* 2008; **246**: 812–22.

5

Staging of hepatocellular carcinoma

Jorge A. Marrero and Hero K. Hussain

When determining the prognosis of patients with solid tumors, tumor staging and tumor grading are important factors to take into account. Tumor staging describes the extent of tumor in the primary organ and throughout the body. Staging is important for planning treatment, estimating prognosis, providing a standardized platform to evaluate new treatments, and comparing the results of different studies [1]. In the majority of solid organ tumors, staging is determined at the time of surgery and by pathological examination of the resected specimen using the Tumor–Node–Metastasis (TNM) classification.

In addition to tumor burden, histological tumor-grading systems have been shown to offer prognostic information on some cancers such as prostate, breast, and kidney [2]. Tumor burden and grade cannot be assessed in most patients with hepatocellular carcinoma (HCC), because only about a third of the patients will undergo surgical therapies and some of these patients may have received local therapies prior to surgery limiting the histological examination.

The presence of underlying liver cirrhosis in patients with HCC adds an important dimension that cannot be ignored when discussing prognosis and treatment for these patients, and it is what differentiates HCC from other solid tumors. The majority of patients with HCC have underlying cirrhosis, and the degree of hepatic dysfunction determines which treatment can be applied [3]. Another important factor in the prognosis of patients with HCC is performance status, although it is not HCC-specific. Performance status has been shown to be an important prognostic factor in HCC [4]. Therefore, the prognosis of patients with HCC will rely not only on tumor burden, but also on hepatic function and performance status.

Before discussing the staging systems, it is important to discuss the natural history of HCC. Traditionally, patients with HCC exceeding the criteria for either transplantation or hepatic resection are all characterized as having non-resectable or non-surgical HCC. However, the outcome of these patients is not uniformly dismal.

Primary Carcinomas of the Liver, ed. Hero K. Hussain and Isaac R. Francis. Published by Cambridge University Press. © Cambridge University Press 2010.

The best study on the natural history of non-surgical HCC was performed on 102 patients who were not eligible to receive radical therapies and were randomized to a non-treatment arm within two studies [5]. The multivariate analysis showed that baseline performance status and the presence of constitutional symptoms, vascular invasion, or extrahepatic spread were independent predictors of survival. The 1-, 2-, and 3-year survival was 80%, 65%, and 50%, respectively, for the 48 patients without these adverse factors (i.e., intermediate-stage patients) and 29%, 16%, and 8%, respectively, for the 54 patients with at least one adverse parameter (i.e., advanced-stage patients). This study has been validated by others [6,7]; therefore, non-surgical HCC can be divided further into advanced stage and intermediate stage, the latter with a less dismal prognosis.

Because only a few patients with HCC are treated with surgery, a pathologic TNM staging cannot always be obtained. Therefore, a radiologic TNM staging classification system has been developed and is currently adopted as the main method for identifying patients who can undergo liver transplantation [8]. This staging system only measures tumor burden on cross-sectional imaging; for example, tumors that are T2N0M0 (single tumor between 2 and 5 cm or three tumors each <3 cm in diameter) get priority points for liver transplantation. The drawbacks of this system are that it does not take into account the presence of underlying liver disease or liver function, and is dependent upon the availability of arterial and delayed phases of contrast-enhanced imaging as well as a radiologist with experience in imaging the cirrhotic liver. More importantly, this system has not been found to be accurate in determining the prognosis of patients with HCC [6].

Several staging systems have been proposed for HCC (see Table 5.1). These include the Okuda [9], BCLC (Barcelona Clinic Liver Cancer) [10], CLIP (Cancer of Liver Italian Program) [11], GRETCH (Groupe d'Etude et de Traitement du Carcinome Hépatocellulaire) [12], CUPI (Chinese University Prognostic Index) [13], and JIS (Japanese Integrated Staging) [14] classification. The CLIP, GRETCH, and CUPI systems were each determined by the results of a multivariate analysis of survival factors in a cohort of patients with HCC, which limits their value for several reasons: First, these studies are applicable only to the population studied, leading to lack of transportability; second, many lack validation in an independent cohort, which is critical for the development of such a system; third, some factors that determine tumor burden, hepatic function, and performance status were not taken into account; and last, they lack a link to treatment. Okuda *et al.* [9] realized that tumor burden and hepatic function were the most important factors that determine prognosis of HCC, but their assessment of tumor burden was crude

Table 5.1 Variables included in seven staging systems for HCC

Staging system	Hepatic function	AFP	Performance status	Tumor staging
Okuda	Ascites, albumin, and bilirubin	No	No	Tumor ≥ or <50% of cross-sectional area of liver
TNM	No	No	No	Number of nodules, tumor size, and presence of PVT and metastasis
CLIP	CTP	< or ≥400 ng/ml	No	Number of nodules, tumor ≥ or <50% area of liver, and PVT
BCLC	CTP	No	Yes	Tumor size, number of nodules, and PVT
CUPI	Bilirubin, ascites, alkaline phosphatase	< or ≥500 ng/ml	Presence of symptoms	TNM
JIS	CTP	No	No	TNM
GRETCH	Bilirubin, alkaline phosphatase	< or ≥35 μg/L	Yes	PVT

CTP, Child–Turcotte–Pugh classification; PVT, portal vein thrombosis.

(tumor occupying more or less than 50% of the liver), and measures of hepatic function included only presence of ascites and measurement of serum albumin and bilirubin.

The JIS uses the Child–Turcotte–Pugh classification for hepatic function and the TNM staging system for the tumor, as determined by the Liver Cancer Study Group of Japan, to assess tumor burden. The JIS has been compared to the BCLC and the CLIP systems in a recent study of 1679 patients in Japan from 1976 through 2003, and has been found to provide better prognostic determination [15]. There are several flaws in this study, including the lack of determination of performance status (an essential aspect of the BCLC system) and the marked difference in the accuracy of assessing tumor burden and treatment options from 1976–1990 and 1991–2003, leading to a biased comparison. A study that compared the JIS with the CLIP system found that the JIS was better at predicting outcome, but there was significant overlap in the treatment offered for each JIS stratum. Moreover, the

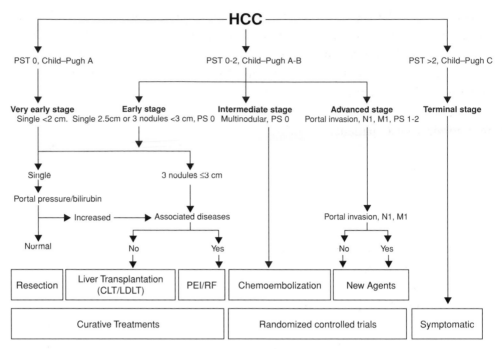

Figure 5.1 The BCLC staging system. Obtained with permission from Llovet et al. [10]. CLT/LDLT, cadaveric liver transplantation/living donor liver transplantation; PEI/RF, percutaneous ethanol injection/radiofrequency thermal ablation.

study did not compare JIS to the BCLC system [16]. No study performed in Japan has compared all the available staging systems for HCC and, to further complicate the situation, a Tokyo prognostic score for HCC was recently developed without being validated in an external cohort of patients [17].

Several studies have shown that the CLIP system has limited value in determining prognosis of patients with HCC [3,18,19]. The problems with the CLIP system are the inability to differentiate the prognosis for patients with stages 1, 2, or 3; the inclusion of alpha-fetoprotein (AFP), which is known to be an unreliable marker for HCC diagnosis; and treatment decisions that often involve overlapping stages. Except for the BCLC system, none of the other prognostic systems provide a treatment algorithm according to tumor stage.

The BCLC system is shown in Figure 5.1. Recent studies compared the BCLC system with the other available systems and found that it is the best at stratifying patients and determining the prognosis of patients with HCC [3,18,19]. In the largest study performed to date, a total of 241 patients was evaluated [6]. The BCLC system was found to be the best at discriminating survival of patients of different stages and had the greatest homogeneity of survival among patients within the same stage. In addition, the BCLC system provided the largest contribution to the Cox model, indicating that it has the best prognostic power for survival compared with other systems. The superiority of the BCLC system over other tumor-staging systems persisted when separate analyses were performed for patients who did not undergo liver transplantation, indicating that it provided better stratification of non-surgical HCC patients at both the intermediate and advanced stages. With regard to transplantation, the T2N0M0 (radiologic TNM) is equal to early-stage BCLC. We believe that the BCLC system had the best prognostication in our study cohort because it included the independent predictors of survival we identified: performance status, measure of hepatic function, and tumor stage (size and portal vein thrombosis). Although the BCLC system does not include treatment as a variable, it has the advantage of stratifying patients into treatment groups and stratifying the nonsurgical group into intermediate and advanced stages. The BCLC system has been endorsed by the American Association for the Study of Liver Diseases (AASLD) in their recent guidelines [3].

At the present time the evidence points toward the BCLC system as the staging system that provides the best prognostic information and linkage to an evidence-based treatment algorithm. It has been externally validated in several populations with all systems included. However, as in all areas of medicine, as our ability to diagnose and treat HCC improves and becomes homogeneous, the validity of the BCLC system and other tumor-staging systems needs to be reevaluated.

REFERENCES

1. Compton CC, Fielding LP, Burgart LJ, *et al*. Prognostic factors in colorectal cancer. College of American Pathologists Consensus Statement 1999. *Arch Pathol Lab Med* 2000; **124**: 979–94.

2. Gleason DF, Veterans Administration Cooperative Urological Research Group. Histologic grading and staging of prostatic carcinoma. In: Tannenbaum M, ed. Urologic pathology: The prostate. Philadelphia: Lea & Febiger, 1977: 171–87.

3. Bruix J and Sherman M. Management of hepatocellular carcinoma. *Hepatology* 2005; **42**: 1208–36.

4. Llovet JM and Bruix J. Early diagnosis and treatment of hepatocellular carcinoma. *Baillieres Best Pract Res Clin Gastroenterol* 2000; **14**: 991–1008.

5. Llovet JM, Bustamante J, Castells A, *et al*. Natural history of untreated nonsurgical hepatocellular carcinoma: Rationale for the design and evaluation of therapeutic trials. *Hepatology* 1999; **29**: 62–7.

6. Marrero JA, Fontana RJ, Barrat A, *et al.* Prognosis of hepatocellular carcinoma: Comparison of 7 staging systems in an American cohort. *Hepatology* 2005; **41**: 707–15.

7. Yeung YP, Lo CM, Liu CL, Wong BC, Fan ST, and Wong J. Natural history of untreated nonsurgical hepatocellular carcinoma. *Am J Gastroenterol* 2005; **100**: 1995–2004.

8. The United Network for Organ Sharing [cited May 20, 2009]. Available from: http://www.unos.org/PoliciesandBylaws2/policies/pdfs/policy_8.pdf

9. Okuda K, Ohtsuki T, Obata H, *et al.* Natural history of hepatocellular carcinoma and prognosis in relation to treatment. Study of 850 patients. *Cancer* 1985; **56**: 918–28.

10. Llovet JM, Bru C, and Bruix J. Prognosis of hepatocellular carcinoma: The BCLC staging classification. *Semin Liver Dis* 1999; **19**: 329–38.

11. The Cancer of the Liver Italian Program (CLIP) Investigators. Prospective validation of the CLIP score: A new prognostic system for patients with cirrhosis and hepatocellular carcinoma. *Hepatology* 2000; **31**: 840–5.

12. Chevret S, Trinchet JC, Mathieu D, Rached AA, Beaugrand M, and Chastang C. For the Groupe d'Etude et de Traitement du Carcinome Hépatocellulaire. A new prognostic classification for predicting survival in patients with hepatocellular carcinoma. *J Hepatol* 1999; **31**: 133–41.

13. Leung TW, Tang AM, Zee B, *et al.* Construction of the Chinese University Prognostic Index for hepatocellular carcinoma and comparison with the TNM staging system, the Okuda staging system, and the Cancer of the Liver Italian Program staging system: A study based on 926 patients. *Cancer* 2002; **94**: 1760–9.

14. Kudo M, Chung H, and Osaki Y. Prognostic staging system for hepatocellular carcinoma (CLIP score): Its value and limitations, and a proposal for a new staging system, the Japan Integrated Staging score (JIS score). *J Gastroenterol* 2003; **38**: 207–15.

15. Toyoda H, Kumada T, Kiriyama S, *et al.* Comparison of the usefulness of three staging systems for hepatocellular carcinoma (CLIP, BCLC, and JIS) in Japan. *Am J Gastroenterol* 2005; **100**: 1764–71.

16. Kudo M, Chung H, Haji S, *et al.* Validation of a new prognostic staging system for hepatocellular carcinoma: The JIS score compared with the CLIP score. *Hepatology* 2004; **40**: 1396–405.

17. Tateishi R, Yoshida H, Shiina S, *et al.* Proposal of a new prognostic model for hepatocellular carcinoma: An analysis of 403 patients. *Gut* 2005; **54**: 419–25.

18. Cillo U, Bassanellos M, Vitale A, *et al.* The critical issue of hepatocellular carcinoma prognostic classification: Which is the best tool available? *J Hepatol* 2004; **40**: 124–31.

19. Huang YH, Chen CH, Chang TT, *et al.* Evaluation of predictive value of CLIP, Okuda, TNM and JIS staging systems for hepatocellular carcinoma patients undergoing surgery. *J Gastroenterol Hepatol* 2005; **20**: 765–71.

6

Surgical treatment of hepatocellular carcinoma: resection and transplantation

Sean Kumer and Shawn J. Pelletier

Hepatocellular carcinoma (HCC) represents approximately 80–90% of primary liver malignancies around the world, and its prevalence parallels that of chronic liver disease [1]. Its incidence peaks between the ages of 50 and 70 years, and it is more common in men than in women. Risk factors include cirrhosis, chronic hepatitis, carcinogens, and inborn errors of metabolism. HCCs can be solitary, multicentric, diffuse, as well as infiltrating. The tumor may invade adjacent vascular structures or metastasize to the lungs, adrenal glands, lymph nodes, or bone. After HCC is diagnosed, the overall survival is poor, with an approximate 50% mortality within the first year following diagnosis. Survival is associated with the size of the tumor, the number of satellite lesions, and overall hepatic function. As a result, high-risk surveillance programs have been initiated in many areas throughout the world to detect early-stage tumors. Furthermore, advancements in imaging have allowed for identification of these malignancies at earlier stages. The end result has allowed for increasingly higher rates of potential cure by either resection or transplantation.

Patients with HCC frequently have underlying cirrhotic liver disease. Hepatic dysfunction and cirrhosis-related portal hypertension, however, can be limiting factors for surgical resection. The first line of therapy for HCC continues to be surgical resection. However, decreased hepatic reserve and portal hypertension make surgical resection in cirrhotic patients increasingly more tenuous and are associated with increased morbidity and mortality. Cirrhotic patients also have a high rate of cancer recurrence [2,3]. Resection can only be performed safely in a subset of patients because many patients present with decompensated cirrhosis, multifocal HCC, or tumors requiring a major resection in the setting of limited hepatic reserve. For patients with decompensated cirrhosis and tumors that have not progressed beyond Tumor–Node–Metastasis (TNM) stage II (i.e., within the Milan criteria of a solitary tumor ≤ 5 cm or up to three lesions each less than

Primary Carcinomas of the Liver, ed. Hero K. Hussain and Isaac R. Francis. Published by Cambridge University Press. © Cambridge University Press 2010.

3 cm without evidence of vascular invasion) [4], the best option may be liver transplantation [5].

For patients with solitary tumors and well-compensated cirrhosis not requiring hepatic resection of four or more segments, the optimal treatment strategy is most often resection, but this strategy remains under intense debate [6]. The major limitation on HCC resection is the presence of cirrhosis. Its absence permits much more extensive hepatic resections to achieve a curative operation. The operative mortality and morbidity are also lower in non-cirrhotic patients than in those with cirrhosis. In the West, approximately 80% of patients with HCC have cirrhosis, whereas in Asia, approximately 68% of patients with HCC have underlying cirrhosis [7]. The 5-year survival after resection of HCC in patients without cirrhosis is approximately 40%, which is similar to the 5-year survival in patients with cirrhosis [7]. Patient selection also greatly influences the survival rate. This has been illustrated by several series reporting that, in selected cirrhotic patients, the 5-year survival rate following resection can be 50–70% [8,9,10,11]. Therefore, preoperative evaluation to determine the extent of fibrosis, the hepatic reserve, the presence of cirrhosis, and the extent of portal hypertension is paramount.

Patient selection

As with any major surgical procedure, the usual preoperative evaluations should be pursued. However, there are specific criteria for those patients with end-stage liver disease. The degree of portal hypertension has been used to help predict the ability of a patient to tolerate resection. Portal hypertension is likely present if esophageal varices or abdominal ascites are present. Also, clinically significant portal hypertension can be suspected if the platelet count is less than 100 000/uL and the patient has splenomegaly [12]. Furthermore, the pressure gradient between the right atrium and the wedged hepatic vein (corrected sinusoidal pressure) can be measured using hepatic vein catheterization. Portal hypertension is defined as corrected sinusoidal pressure greater than or equal to 10 mm Hg.

In addition to the assessment for portal hypertension, functional hepatic reserve must also be evaluated. Normal bilirubin levels and coagulation studies usually signify an adequate hepatic reserve to tolerate resection. In Japan, indocyanine green retention has been used to determine the physiologically tolerable extent of resection with less than or equal to 20% retention after 15 minutes denoting adequate reserve [13].

In patients with a normal total bilirubin and no portal hypertension, the risk for decompensation is low and a 5-year survival rate greater than 70% can be achieved in resected HCC patients [14,15]. In the short term, despite an initially increased operative risk, patients with cirrhosis who have adequate hepatic reserve may fare as well as patients who do not have cirrhosis [7]. More recently, the Model for End-Stage Liver Disease (MELD) has been used to predict postsurgical outcome in patients with cirrhosis [16].

Preoperative evaluation of cirrhotics has traditionally included determination of Child–Turcotte–Pugh (CTP) classification [17,18]. However, there is a wide variation in the extent of liver disease found in patients with CTP Class A cirrhosis. Patients with CTP Class A cirrhosis may have portal hypertension, mild elevations in bilirubin, or fluid retention, all of which can be features of advanced disease [19,20]. CTP classification alone does not accurately predict which patients will tolerate surgical resection [21]. The study by Befeler et al. [21] suggested that a MELD score greater than 14 may replace CTP Class C as a more accurate predictor of poor outcomes following general abdominal procedures. MELD has been used specifically as a predictor of hepatic resection outcomes in patients with HCC [16]. The study by Teh et al. [16] suggested that hepatic resection in cirrhotic patients with HCC be limited to scores of less than 8 and those with scores greater than 9 be considered for other therapies. Conversely, the predictive value of the MELD system does not hold true for non-cirrhotic patients undergoing HCC resections [22]. Overall, the goal is to be able to resect early-stage HCC prior to the progression of disease, and perform transplantations for those patients who have HCC within the Milan criteria.

Controversy still remains regarding downstaging previously unresectable and untransplantable patients with modalities such as transarterial chemoembolization (TACE) and radiofrequency ablation (RFA) to qualify them for resection or, more likely, orthotopic liver transplantation. No significant effect on mortality has been described for RFA or TACE when performed as a bridge to transplantation for patients who undergo transplantation within 6 months of listing [23,24].

Preoperative imaging

Preoperative imaging is essential in developing a plan of care for the patient. Depending on the condition of the patient, the plan of care will be modified. In general, a healthier patient with early-stage HCC will most likely be eligible for an operative plan with curative intent via liver transplantation or resection. Other patients may receive locoregional therapy (including RFA, TACE, or yttrium-90–labeled glass beads) either as a bridge to transplantation or as treatment prior to chemotherapy and/or radiation. For instance, the proximity of the lesion(s) to vasculature will alter plans for RFA as well as for resection because RFA may not be an efficacious alternative and resection plans may have to be altered or discontinued secondary to the necessity for extended resections. Nonetheless, anatomical considerations are a priority in operative planning as well as in preparation for RFA and TACE procedures.

Operative intervention

Resection

As mentioned previously, patient selection determines whether a patient will tolerate a resection. Surgical resection is clearly the recommended therapy in those patients without cirrhosis. As a general rule, resection candidacy is primarily limited to CTP Class A cirrhotics and to cirrhotics with a MELD score less than 8. Hepatic resection in these physiologically tenuous patients is most often limited to wedge resections when at all possible. Anatomical resections are not always tolerated, but occasionally certain patients will qualify. Anatomically favorable lesions include those closest to the liver's surface and not juxtaposed to major hepatic vasculature. As mentioned earlier, the 5-year survival after HCC resection in non-cirrhotic patients is approximately 40%. This survival rate is commensurate with resections in cirrhotic patients, but the average size of resected tumors in non-cirrhotic patients tends to be larger than in cirrhotic patients. If careful preoperative screening is performed, the 5-year survival after resection in cirrhotic patients can exceed 50%.

For patients with compensated cirrhosis who are eligible for resection, the least amount of liver possible should be resected. In most cases, the procedure will involve a wedge or a segmental anatomic resection according to Couinaud criteria. With modern technology, segmental resections in selected cirrhotic patients can safely be performed without the need for blood transfusions or significant morbidity or mortality [13,14,25]. Neoadjuvant therapies such as TACE prior to resection do not appear beneficial in decreasing tumor size and the size of the needed resection [26]. A left hepatic lobectomy may be possible in selected cirrhotic patients; however, a right hepatic lobectomy is more likely to result in postoperative liver failure as it constitutes the majority of the hepatic parenchyma. Volumetric analysis of the liver to be resected is useful for more extensive resections [13]. However, there are minimal data that help to determine a safe resection based on the volume of the remnant functional liver in cirrhotic patients. When an extensive resection is anticipated and hepatic reserve is questionable, portal vein embolization (PVE) of the involved hepatic lobe can be performed several weeks preoperatively to induce compensatory hypertrophy in the unaffected lobe (surgical remnant) [27,28]. However, no randomized studies have been performed to confirm that PVE is beneficial, particularly in patients with cirrhosis. There are disadvantages in the delay that PVE requires prior to resection, PVE may induce hepatic failure, and it may induce malignant hepatocytes to proliferate as well.

The general tenet of ensuring a clear surgical margin in resections of HCC is controversial. Larger HCC tumors often present with satellite tumors surrounding the dominant lesion. Whereas some reports suggest that surgical margins of less than 1 cm are associated with higher rates of intrahepatic recurrence, other reports have not confirmed that contention [29,30,31]. Moreover, the utility of a 1 cm margin has been challenged. Frequent detection of synchronous tumors in the pathology specimen suggests that recurrence near the surgical site may be due to an undetected synchronous tumor, an incomplete resection, or failure to include all satellite lesions. Overall, a negative pathological margin is generally considered acceptable.

Transplantation

Liver transplantation for HCC in the 1980s had poor outcomes, with HCC recurrence and subsequent survival being unacceptably dismal. Since the publication of the Milan criteria by Mazzaferro et al. [4], HCC meeting these criteria has been the standard for liver transplantation. The posttransplant survival in HCC patients with tumor within the Milan criteria is commensurate with other liver recipients without cancer. Liver transplantation has the advantage of allowing for wide resection margins of the primary HCC as well as satellite tumors, removal of the remaining cirrhotic liver where metachronous tumors may occur, and return to normal liver function. The end result is that the malignant potential of remaining cirrhotic liver is removed, normal liver function is restored, and portal hypertension is eliminated. The trade-off is that there is the need for lifelong immunosuppression and its associated sequelae.

The Milan criteria clearly define that either a solitary tumor less than or equal to 5 cm in diameter or multifocal HCC with three or fewer tumors each measuring less than or equal to 3 cm in diameter is associated with improved outcomes following liver transplantation. The 4-year actuarial and disease-free survival in patients with HCC meeting the Milan criteria was 83% and 75%, respectively [4]. More liberal criteria for transplantation, including the University of California San Francisco criteria (one lesion <8 cm or three lesions <5 cm with total tumor diameter <8 cm or five lesions <3 cm with a total tumor diameter <8 cm) [32], have been applied in an attempt to identify more patients with acceptable outcomes following transplantation; however, none has gained universal acceptance.

In February 2002, the deceased-donor liver allocation system in the United States was modified to use severity of illness as determined by the MELD score rather than waiting time. Candidates with HCC within Milan criteria are given an increased-exception MELD score (currently 22 points), so that more than half of the liver candidates with HCC meeting Milan criteria are transplanted within 90 days of listing. If patients with HCC have not received a transplant within 3 months, an additional 3 points are awarded for the theoretical 10% increase in HCC-related mortality while on the waiting list. Suspicious tumors less than 2 cm in diameter have been found to have a relatively high false-positive rate for HCC on imaging and have generally shown a slow progression of tumor growth. Subsequently, candidates with a single suspicious nodule or even biopsy-proven HCC less than 2 cm are not given an exception MELD score. Most candidates with HCC have relatively low MELD scores (without the HCC exception points) when compared to other liver transplant candidates who usually have hepatic decompensation as the cause of their listing. Those HCC patients without the added exception score, because of tumors beyond Milan criteria or with a solitary nodule less than 2 cm in diameter, are effectively excluded from having a liver allocated from the deceased-donor waiting list. Despite being counterintuitive to oncologic principles, the rule is that candidates with small tumors essentially need to wait for deceased-donor transplantation until the tumor size has increased to greater than or equal to 2 cm in diameter. Tumors less than 2 cm in diameter, as a result, are often treated with other therapeutic options including RFA, TACE, or living donor liver transplantation.

When considering all candidates listed for liver transplantation, approximately 20% will die or otherwise be removed from the waiting list because of becoming too ill or from progression of their tumor [14]. As a result, bridging strategies have been developed prior to transplantation. These are principally RFA and TACE. For those patients who undergo transplantation within 6 months of listing, pretransplant therapies such as TACE or RFA have not demonstrated a significant effect on survival [23,24]. The availability of a living donor essentially eliminates the risk of mortality while on the waiting list. Living-donor transplantation remains a reasonable option for those HCC patients within the Milan criteria as well as those with a solitary tumor less than 2 cm in diameter.

In summary, ever-increasing improvements in imaging and screening for HCC in patients with cirrhosis and chronic viral hepatitis have allowed for an increased number of patients to be identified with early-stage tumors that would be amenable to surgical resection or, ultimately, liver transplantation. For non-cirrhotic patients, surgical resection is the established standard of care, if at all feasible. For patients with compensated cirrhosis, adequate hepatic reserve, and little to no clinical evidence of portal hypertension, surgical resection may also be the optimal therapy. For patients with tumors within the Milan criteria and with evidence of cirrhotic decompensation, multifocal disease, or disease burden requiring extensive resection, liver transplantation is the treatment of choice.

REFERENCES

1. Martin P. Hepatocellular carcinoma: Risk factors and natural history. *Liver Transpl Surg* 1998; **4**: 87–91.

2. Yamamoto J, Kosuge T, Takayama T, *et al.* Recurrence of hepatocellular carcinoma after surgery. *Br J Surg* 1996; **83**: 1219–22.

3. Poon RT, Fan ST, Lo CM, Liu CL, and Wong J. Intrahepatic recurrence after curative resection of hepatocellular carcinoma. Long-term results of treatment and prognostic factors. *Ann Surg* 1999; **229**: 216–22.

4. Mazzaferro V, Regalia E, Doci R, *et al.* Liver transplantation for the treatment of small hepatocellular carcinomas in patients with cirrhosis. *N Engl J Med* 1996; **334**: 693–9.

5. Llovet JM, Burroughs A, and Bruix J. Hepatocellular carcinoma. *Lancet* 2003; **362**: 1907–17.

6. Llovet JM, Bruix J, and Gores GJ. Surgical resection versus transplantation for early hepatocellular carcinoma: Clues for the best strategy. *Hepatology* 2000; **31**: 1019–21.

7. Vauthey JN, Klimstra D, Franceschi D, *et al.* Factors affecting long-term outcome after hepatic resection for hepatocellular carcinoma. *Am J Surg* 1995; **169**: 28–34; discussion 34–5.

8. Arii S, Yamaoka Y, Futagawa S, *et al.* Results of surgical and nonsurgical treatment for small-sized hepatocellular carcinomas: A retrospective and nationwide survey in Japan. The Liver Cancer Study Group of Japan. *Hepatology* 2000; **32**: 1224–9.

9. Takayama T, Makuuchi M, Hirohashi S, *et al.* Early hepatocellular carcinoma as an entity with a high rate of surgical cure. *Hepatology* 1998; **28**: 1241–6.

10. Fong Y, Sun RL, Jarnagin W, and Blumgart LH. An analysis of 412 cases of hepatocellular carcinoma at a Western center. *Ann Surg* 1999; **229**: 790–9; discussion 799–800.

11. Grazi GL, Ercolani G, Pierangeli F, *et al.* Improved results of liver resection for hepatocellular carcinoma on cirrhosis give the procedure added value. *Ann Surg* 2001; **234**: 71–8.

12. Bruix J and Sherman M. Management of hepatocellular carcinoma. *Hepatology* 2005; **42**: 1208–36.

13. Torzilli G, Makuuchi M, Inoue K, *et al.* No-mortality liver resection for hepatocellular carcinoma in cirrhotic and noncirrhotic patients: Is there a way? A prospective analysis of our approach. *Arch Surg* 1999; **134**: 984–92.

14. Llovet JM, Fuster J, and Bruix J. Intention-to-treat analysis of surgical treatment for early hepatocellular carcinoma: Resection versus transplantation. *Hepatology* 1999; **30**: 1434–40.

15. Bruix J, Castells A, Bosch J, *et al.* Surgical resection of hepatocellular carcinoma in cirrhotic patients: Prognostic value of preoperative portal pressure. *Gastroenterology* 1996; **111**: 1018–22.

16. Teh SH, Christien J, Donohue J, *et al.* Hepatic resection of hepatocellular carcinoma in patients with cirrhosis: Model of end-stage liver disease (MELD) score predicts perioperative mortality. *J Gastroint Surg* 2005; **9**: 1207–15.

17. Pugh RNH, Murray-Lyon IM, Dawson JL, Pietroni MC, and Williams R. Transection of the oesophagus for bleeding oesophageal varices. *Br J Surg* 1973; **60**: 646–9.

18. Child CG and Turcotte JG. Surgery and portal hypertension. In: Child CG, ed. *The liver and portal hypertension.* Philadelphia: Saunders, 1964: 50–64.

19. D'Amico G, Morabito A, Pagliaro L, and Marubini E. Survival and prognostic indicators in compensated and decompensated cirrhosis. *Dig Dis Sci* 1986; **31**: 468–75.

20. Gines P, Quintero E, Arroyo V, *et al.* Compensated cirrhosis: Natural history and prognostic factors. *Hepatology* 1987; **7**: 122–8.

21. Befeler AS, Palmer DE, Hoffman M, Longo W, Solomon H, and Di Bisceglie AM. The safety of intra-abdominal surgery in patients with cirrhosis. *Arch Surg* 2005; **140**: 650–4.

22. Teh SH, Sheppard BC, Schwartz J, and Orloff SL. Model of end-stage liver disease score fails to predict perioperative outcome after hepatic resection for hepatocellular carcinoma in patients without cirrhosis. *Am J Surg* 2008; **195**: 697–701.

23. Porrett PM, Peterman H, Rosen M, *et al.* Lack of benefit of pre-transplant locoregional hepatic therapy for hepatocellular cancer in the current MELD era. *Liver Transpl* 2006; **12**: 665–73.

24. Shiffman ML, Brown RS, Jr., Olthoff KM, *et al.* Living donor liver transplantation: Summary of a conference at The National Institutes of Health. *Liver Transpl* 2002; **8**: 174–88.

25. Rees M, Plant G, Wells J, and Bygrave S. One hundred and fifty hepatic resections: Evolution of technique towards bloodless surgery. *Br J Surg* 1996; **83**: 1526–9.

26. Yamasaki S, Hasegawa H, Kinoshita H, *et al.* A prospective randomized trial of the preventive effect of pre-operative transcatheter arterial embolization against recurrence of hepatocellular carcinoma. *Jpn J Cancer Res* 1996; **87**: 206–11.

27. Tanaka H, Hirohashi K, Kubo S, Shuto T, Higaki I, and Kinoshita H. Preoperative portal vein embolization improves prognosis after right hepatectomy for hepatocellular carcinoma in patients with impaired hepatic function. *Br J Surg* 2000; **87**: 879–82.

28. Farges O, Belghiti J, Kianmanesh R, *et al.* Portal vein embolization before right hepatectomy: Prospective clinical trial. *Ann Surg* 2003; **237**: 208–17.

29. Belghiti J, Panis Y, Farges O, Benhamou JP, and Fekete F. Intrahepatic recurrence after resection of hepatocellular carcinoma complicating cirrhosis. *Ann Surg* 1991; **214**: 114–17.

30. Chen MF, Hwang TL, Jeng LB, Wang CS, Jan YY, and Chen SC. Postoperative recurrence of hepatocellular carcinoma. Two hundred five consecutive patients who underwent hepatic resection in 15 years. *Arch Surg* 1994; **129**: 738–42.

31. Arii S, Tanaka J, Yamazoe Y, *et al.* Predictive factors for intrahepatic recurrence of hepatocellular carcinoma after partial hepatectomy. *Cancer* 1992; **69**: 913–19.

32. Yao FY. Expanded criteria for hepatocellular carcinoma: Down-staging with a view to liver transplantation–yes. *Semin Liver Dis* 2006; **26**: 239–47.

7

Non-surgical treatment of hepatocellular carcinoma

7.1 Regional therapies for treatment of intermediate-stage hepatocellular carcinoma

a. Transarterial chemoembolization

Venkat N. Krishnamurthy

Hepatocellular carcinoma (HCC) incidence is increasing worldwide [1,2]. Without treatment, the prognosis is poor and the 5-year survival rate is less than 5% [3,4]. Surgical resection, liver transplantation, and percutaneous ablation are the only effective treatments that offer improved survival and long-term cure [5,6,7]. However, only 15–30% of patients with HCC are surgical candidates at initial presentation because of tumor extension, multiplicity of tumor foci, and associated advanced liver cirrhosis [8]. When the tumor is unresectable, a variety of other locoregional treatments are offered to improve the quality and duration of life, such as transarterial chemoembolization (TACE), systemic chemotherapy, and radiation therapy. Among these, TACE has been in use since the mid-1970s and has a proven survival benefit [9,10,11,12].

This chapter discusses the rationale, the technique and protocols, the patient selection criteria, and the risks and benefits of TACE. Current trends toward multimodality treatment are also discussed.

Vascular anatomy of the liver

The liver receives dual blood supply; approximately one-third from the hepatic artery and the remaining two-thirds from the portal vein. The arterial supply to the liver usually comes from the celiac artery via the common hepatic artery that branches into the gastroduodenal and proper hepatic arteries (Figure 7.1a.1). The proper hepatic artery then branches into right and left hepatic arteries, which in turn follow the segmental pattern defined by Couinaud's segmental anatomy [13].

Primary Carcinomas of the Liver, ed. Hero K. Hussain and Isaac R. Francis. Published by Cambridge University Press. © Cambridge University Press 2010.

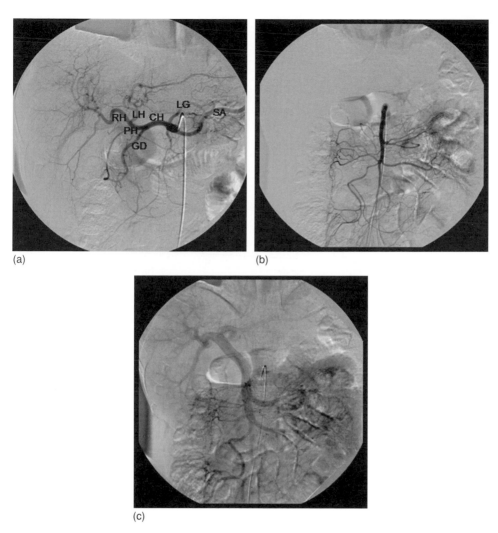

Figure 7.1a.1 (a–c) Vascular anatomy of the liver. (a): Digital subtraction celiac arteriogram demonstrates classical division into common hepatic (CH), left gastric (LG), and splenic arteries (SA). The common hepatic artery divides into gastroduodenal (GD) and proper hepatic (PH) arteries. The proper hepatic artery gives rise to the right hepatic (RH) and left hepatic (LH) arteries. (b and c): Indirect portovenogram obtained during TACE shows patency and flow direction in the portal vein. This is obtained by following a superior mesenteric artery injection (b) through the venous phase (c).

Accessory or replaced hepatic arteries occur, each in 5–15% of patients [14]. Common variations include accessory or replaced left hepatic artery from left gastric artery, accessory or replaced right hepatic artery from superior mesenteric artery, and completely replaced hepatic artery from superior mesenteric artery (Figure 7.1a.2). The right hepatic artery is aberrant in origin in 26% of cases

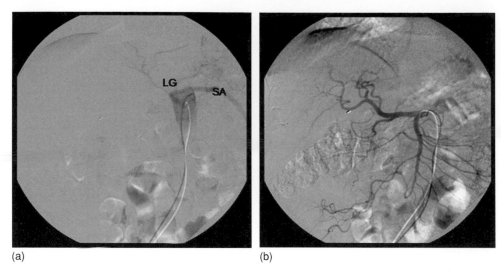

(a)   (b)

Figure 7.1a.2 (a and b) Variant vascular anatomy. (a): Celiac arteriogram shows only splenic (SA) and left gastric (LG) arteries. (b): Superior mesenteric arteriogram shows a completely replaced hepatic artery.

(replaced, 18%; accessory, 8%), and the left hepatic artery is aberrant in origin in 27% (replaced, 15.5%; accessory, 11.5%) [15]. Recognizing the variant anatomy is important for two reasons: The vascular anatomy can make the procedure technically challenging, and the blood supply to neighboring vital organs may result in non-target embolization.

Rationale for transarterial chemoembolization

The TACE procedure involves administration of a mixture of cytotoxic drugs and iodized oil into the hepatic artery supplying the tumor, followed by embolization of the artery to attain ischemia. This achieves three important goals: Deliver a highly concentrated dose of chemotherapy to tumor cells, prolong the contact time between the chemotherapeutic agents and the cancer cells, and minimize systemic toxicity. Effective chemoembolization of hepatic tumors is possible by following different mechanisms:

1. At the very early stages, HCC is not highly vascularized and receives its blood supply from both the hepatic artery and the portal vein. When the tumor becomes more than 2 cm in size, the hepatic artery supply constitutes almost 95% of the total blood supply [16]. This allows targeting treatment of HCC through the hepatic artery.

2. The portal vein provides more than 75% of the normal blood supply allowing for effective hepatic arterial embolization without causing significant liver infarction and dysfunction.
3. Advances in endovascular techniques allow superselective placement of catheters (even in the presence of aberrant vessels or a collateral blood supply) for safe and effective delivery of chemotherapeutic agents to hepatic tumors.
4. When injected into the hepatic artery, iodized oil (Ethiodol; Savage Laboratories, Melville, NY) is known to preferentially flow toward the HCC. The mechanism of oil accumulation in the tumor is not fully understood, but it is likely secondary to the siphoning effect of a vascular tumor. Intraarterially injected oil is well known to demonstrate preferential flow toward vascular tumors. After they accumulate, they remain in the neovasculature and extravascular spaces of the HCC. This makes Ethiodol an effective vehicle for delivering chemotherapy. Ethiodol is as an embolic agent that causes tumor ischemia. In summary, the iodized oil has three important properties: tumor-seeking, drug-carrying, and embolic effect.
5. The chemotherapeutic agents (cisplatin, doxorubicin, and mitomycin C) used in TACE procedures are all metabolized rapidly by the liver resulting in a significant (10- to 100-fold) difference in its concentration between the intrahepatic and systemic circulations. This allows very high doses of these agents to be delivered to the tumor bed with significantly reduced systemic toxicity [17,18].
6. Hepatic artery embolization results in ischemic necrosis of the tumor. There is ischemia-induced failure of the transmembrane pumps in tumor cells [19] that results in increased absorption and retention of chemotherapeutic drugs. Thus ischemia prolongs the duration of contact of chemotherapeutic agents with tumor cells, thereby increasing the cytotoxic effect [20].

Transarterial chemoembolization procedure

Preprocedure evaluation

The two most important factors that affect the decision to offer TACE are the stage of HCC and the type and extent of the underlying liver disease (Table 7.1a.1). The diagnosis of HCC is first established either directly with tissue biopsy or indirectly by means of imaging. Focused clinical and laboratory evaluation is performed to assess severity of underlying liver disease and the stage of HCC. Multiphasic contrast-enhanced magnetic resonance imaging (MRI) or computed tomography (CT) of the liver is performed, as well as CT of the chest and a bone scan to assess

Table 7.1a.1 Key aspects in the preprocedural evaluation for TACE

A. Most important factors that affect the decision to offer TACE:
1. Type and severity of the underlying chronic liver disease
2. Stage of HCC

B. Most important components of evaluation:
1. Establishing the diagnosis of HCC – Biopsy, combination of clinical features/tumor marker (AFP) and imaging characteristics of the liver mass
2. Detailed clinical history and physical examination
3. Laboratory evaluation to document tumor markers and determine severity of chronic liver disease. Classification of severity of cirrhosis according to the CTP system (Class A, B, and C)
4. Imaging evaluation with MRI or CT to assess the stage of HCC

the stage of HCC and ensure the absence of metastatic disease and any comorbid disease.

Patient selection criteria

The indication and contraindications for TACE remain controversial, and it can be somewhat difficult to determine which patient and/or tumor characteristics best predict survival benefit [12,21]. TACE is usually offered when patients are not eligible for curative options such as surgical resection or transplantation. Guidelines for selecting patients for TACE are detailed in Table 7.1a.2. In general, patients with smaller tumors and well-preserved liver functions are better candidates [22,23]. Patients with poor baseline liver function and large tumors benefit least from TACE [22,24].

TACE is not feasible in patients with contraindications to the arterial procedure (uncorrectable coagulopathy, severe atherosclerotic disease precluding access to the hepatic artery) or to the administration of doxorubicin (serum bilirubin >85.5 mmol/L, leukocyte count <3000/mm^3, or cardiac ejection fraction <50%).

Portal vein thrombosis is not an absolute contraindication for TACE [25,26]. The procedure can safely be carried out if hepatopetal flow is demonstrated in periportal collaterals and by performing superselective or segmental rather than lobar chemoembolization (Figure 7.1a.3).

HCC patients with biliary obstruction require extra precautions to avoid causing biliary necrosis in the obstructed segment(s) of the liver, which may result in abscess formation; therefore, percutaneous or endoscopic biliary drainage must

Table 7.1a.2 Patient selection criteria for TACE

Good Candidates:
- Tumor diameter <8 cm
- Minimal replacement of liver by tumor tissue (<5%)
- Higher degree of Ethiodol retention by tumor tissue

Poor Candidates:
- Tumor diameter >10 cm
- Diffuse tumor growth pattern
- Infiltrating tumor
- Presence of more than nine tumors within the liver
- Albumin levels <35 gL

Very Poor Candidates:
- More than 50% replacement of the liver by tumor
- Advanced liver disease (CTP Class C)
- Active gastrointestinal bleeding
- Hepatic encephalopathy
- Hepatofugal flow in the portal vein
- Renal failure

TACE of Questionable Value:
- Severe comorbidities
- Extrahepatic metastasis
- Elderly patients (>75 years)

be performed prior to the TACE procedure. The TACE protocol should also be altered (decrease degree of embolization) to avoid biliary ischemia and necrosis [27]. Prior biliary reconstructive surgery (biliary-enteric bypass) increases the risk for development of liver abscesses [28]. In such cases, prophylactic treatment with intravenous broad-spectrum antibiotics is recommended.

Transarterial chemoembolization procedural steps

Informed consent explaining the risks and benefits of TACE should be obtained in all patients. Vigorous hydration with intravenous fluids (normal saline solution at a rate of 200–300 mL/h), prophylactic antibiotics (1 g of cefazolin, 500 mg of metronidazole), and antiemetics (24 mg of ondansetron hydrochloride, 10 mg of decadron, and 50 mg of diphenhydramine) are usually administered.

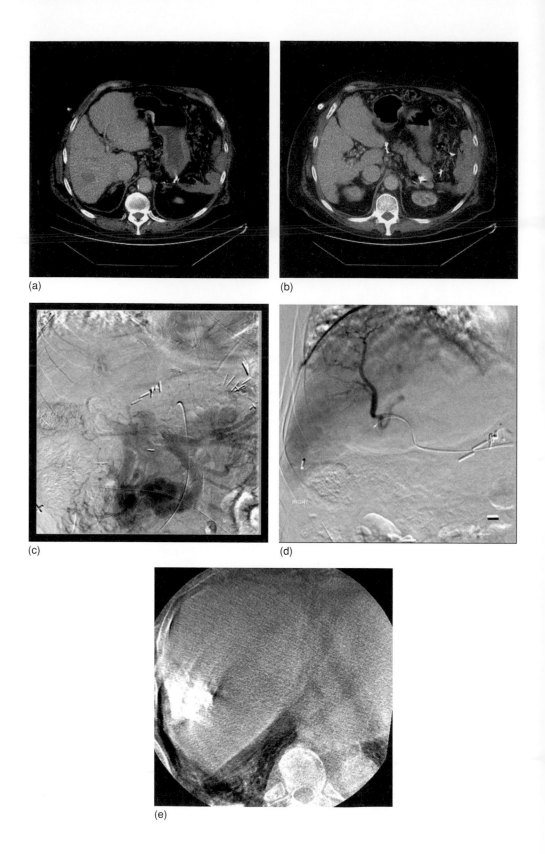

(a)

(b)

(c)

(d)

(e)

A diagnostic visceral (celiac and superior mesenteric) arteriogram with or without aortography is first performed via a common femoral artery approach. When severe aortoiliac occlusive disease precludes the femoral approach, a brachial arterial access may be used. After studying the arterial anatomy, the catheter is advanced into the hepatic artery that feeds the tumor. Newer techniques such as CT angiography can help to ensure that the tumor-containing region of the liver is targeted [29].

Lobar TACE is recommended for patients with multiple or large diffuse tumors (Figure 7.1a.4). Patients with unifocal tumors are best treated with segmental TACE (Figure 7.1a.3). Whole-liver TACE should not be performed because of the potential serious injury to the organ.

Chemotherapy and embolization protocols

No standard intraarterial chemotherapy protocol has been developed. The most common single agent used is doxorubicin (Adriamycin; Pharmacia Upjohn, Kalamazoo, MI), and the most common combination regimen is a mixture of 100 mg of cisplatin (Bristol-Myers Squibb, Princeton, NJ), 50 mg of doxorubicin, and 10 mg of mitomycin C (Bedford Laboratories, Bedford, OH) mixed in 10 mL of water-soluble contrast material (Omnipaque; Winthrop Pharmaceuticals, New York, NY). The chemotherapy solution is emulsified in an equivalent volume of Ethiodol. It is generally recommended not to inject more than 20 mL of Ethiodol for each session of lobar TACE due to the risk of liver failure and pulmonary embolism [30].

A variety of embolic agents have been used, such as gelatin sponge powder and pledgets (Gelfoam; Upjohn, Kalamazoo, MI), 150- to 250 μm size polyvinyl alcohol (PVA) particles (Target Therapeutics, Fremont, CA), Ethiodol, and autologous blood clots. Gelfoam is a temporary embolic agent with recanalization occurring within 2–6 weeks, whereas PVA particles are permanent embolic agents.

Figure 7.1a.3 (a–e) TACE in a 70-year-old male with chronic portal venous thrombosis. (a): CT scan of the liver shows a low attenuation tumor in the right lobe. Biopsy confirmed HCC. (b): CT scan at the level of hepatic hilum shows multiple venous collaterals replacing the portal vein indicating chronic portal venous thrombosis and cavernous transformation. (c): Indirect portovenogram (delayed venous phase after a superior mesenteric arteriogram) shows large mesenteric varices, absent main portal vein and small periportal collaterals. (d): Superselective chemoembolization of segment 7 was performed. (e): DynaCT image (DynaCT; Siemens AG, Berlin, Germany) of liver obtained during the TACE procedure shows the distribution of the chemotherapy–Ethiodol mixture to be limited to the tumor in segment 7.

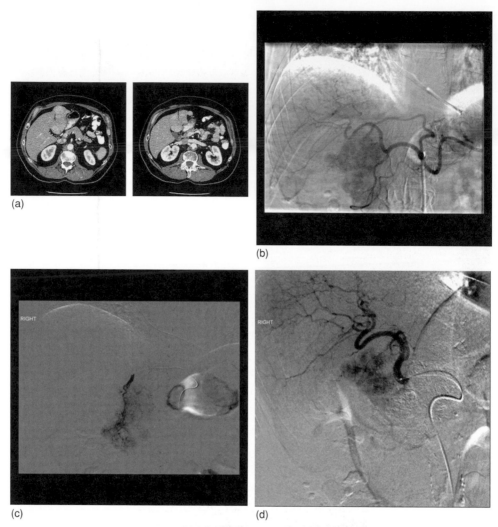

Figure 7.1a.4 (a–g) TACE in a 56-year-old male with a large left lobe HCC. **(a):** Serial axial contrast CT images show a large enhancing tumor replacing most of the left lobe of liver. **(b):** Celiac arteriogram during the TACE procedure shows a large hypervascular mass, predominantly supplied by left hepatic artery. **(c and d):** Left lobar TACE was performed after selective cannulation of the left hepatic artery (c) and segment 4 branches (d). **(e and f):** Spot radiograph (e) and CT scan (f) of the liver obtained at the completion of TACE shows distribution of the chemotherapy–Ethiodol mixture throughout the tumor. **(g):** Follow-up CT scan 1 year after the procedure shows Ethiodol accumulation in the tumor and significantly decreased size of tumor. No enhancement seen to suggest residual or recurrent tumor.

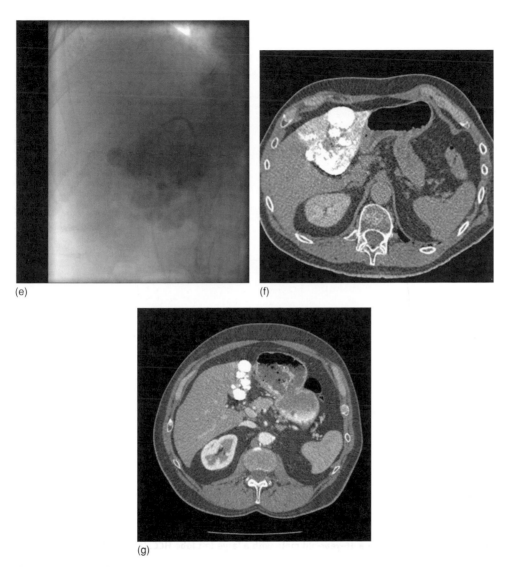

(e)

(f)

(g)

Figure 7.1a.4 (cont.)

Controversy surrounds the method of delivery: Some interventionalists favor mixing the particles in a slurry (thin paste or semifluid mixture) with the chemotherapeutic drugs, whereas others prefer to administer the particles after delivering chemotherapy. Studies have shown that by embolizing the tumor-feeding vessel only after the entire dose of chemotherapy is delivered, injectable volumes of chemotherapy and long-term arterial patency could be significantly improved, thereby improving the efficacy of TACE [31].

Follow-up and retreatment protocols

Clinical follow-up and laboratory studies are usually performed at 1–3 weeks after the procedure. Early repeat imaging (0–14 days) after the procedure helps to determine the adequacy of treatment. The procedure is considered successful when there is greater than 50% lipiodol uptake in the tumor on CT (Figure 7.1a.4F). When the uptake is less than 50%, repeat MRI or CT scan is performed in 6–8 weeks; if the size of the enhancing tumor is reduced, repeat TACE may be considered. Patients with bilobar disease may return for TACE of the other lobe in 4 weeks. Routine follow-up imaging is usually performed at intervals of 3, 6, and 12 months and then yearly.

Indications for retreatment after initial successful TACE remain controversial. Although most centers perform repeat TACE as needed (documented residual or recurrent tumor on follow-up imaging or increasing alpha-fetoprotein [AFP]), recent randomized trials [10,32] recommend repeat TACE at regular intervals of 2–3 months to achieve sustained response.

Recent advances – drug-eluting beads

Strategies to improve the efficacy of TACE are increasing by increasing the intensity and duration of contact between tumor cells and chemotherapeutic drugs, and by decreasing the systemic toxicity through inducing increased retention of the chemotherapeutic agent within the tumor. This can be achieved by loading the embolization particles with chemotherapeutic drugs and allowing for slower release of these drugs [33]. These are known as drug-eluting beads (DEBs) (Angio-Dynamics, Queensbury, NY). DEBs are deformable microspheres produced from a biocompatible PVA hydrogel that has been modified with sulfonate groups for the controlled loading and delivery of chemotherapeutic drugs. These are commercially available under the trade name of DC (or precision) beads (in Europe) or LC beads (in the United States). The DC or precision beads are preloaded with doxorubicin (37.5 mg/mL), whereas the LC beads are loaded in the hospital pharmacy (maximum dose of doxorubicin 75 mg/m^2 or 150 mg per TACE session). Recent studies have shown that TACE with DEBs increases tumor response, reduces systemic toxicity, and improves survival in unresectable HCC [34,35].

Safety of the transarterial chemoembolization procedure

Complications

Reported complication rates vary greatly. Postembolization syndrome is common, consisting of pain, fever, nausea and vomiting, and abdominal discomfort or pain

[36]. It is seen in almost all patients to some degree. Narcotics, antiemetics, and acetaminophen are given to relieve symptoms.

Severe adverse events are less common (3–4%) and 30-day mortality rates range from 1 to 4% [37]. Severe adverse events include hepatic insufficiency or infarction, hepatic abscess and/or generalized septicemia, tumor rupture, bile duct injury, cholecystitis, upper gastrointestinal tract bleeding, pulmonary embolism, pancytopenia, splenic infarction, and spinal embolization. Of these events, the most frequent and serious complication is hepatic insufficiency [38]. Non-target embolization of organs other than the liver and renal failure are rare [37,39,40].

Transarterial chemoembolization in high-risk candidates

Patients are generally considered to be at high risk for TACE if they have one or more of the following: severe hepatic insufficiency (serum bilirubin >2 mg/dL, low serum albumin <3.5 mg/dL, Child–Turcotte–Pugh (CTP) class B or C), multifocal tumor, portal venous flow diversion and/or occlusion (caused by a transjugular intrahepatic portosystemic shunt, portal venous occlusion/thrombosis), or biliary obstruction [38,41,42]. Recent studies have shown that TACE in such patients does not result in higher morbidity or mortality [43,44], and recommend that patient selection be based on the extent of disease and that segmental TACE be used whenever possible.

Efficacy of transarterial chemoembolization

There are numerous studies reporting the efficacy of TACE, but it is difficult to compare these studies because of the significant differences in the patient selection criteria, TACE techniques, and end points as a measure of success. Given the short life expectancy of patients with HCC, patient survival is the most important measure of success [45]. However, most studies use imaging response as a measure of success [46,47,48,49].

A number of retrospective and well-designed case–control studies have shown a survival benefit in patients treated with TACE compared with untreated patients [50,51] or historical control subjects [50,52]. Matsui et al. reported survival rates as high as 100% at 1 year and 53% at 5 years in patients with small HCC treated with TACE [53]. In patients with larger HCC (<50% of the liver), Vetter et al. reported a 1-year survival rate of 59% in patients treated with TACE and 0% in untreated control subjects [54]. Two recently published randomized controlled trials (RCTs) conclusively support the survival benefit from TACE, compared to non-active treatment [10,32]. Metaanalyses of RCTs also suggest that, in patients with unresectable HCC, TACE significantly improved the overall 2-year survival compared with non-active treatments [45].

Combinations of transarterial chemoembolization and other treatments

Transarterial chemoembolization as neoadjuvant and adjuvant treatment

TACE was advocated to improve surgical resectability, decrease dropout rates from the liver transplantation waiting list, and improve survival when performed after surgical resection [55]. However, metaanalyses and results of RCTs do not support these benefits [56,57,58,59].

Combination of transarterial chemoembolization and percutaneous ethanol injection

Combining TACE and percutaneous ethanol injection is proposed to have synergistic benefit. The hypothesis is that TACE induces tumor necrosis, which then potentiates the diffusion of ethanol through the tumor. RCTs and non-randomized studies have documented significantly improved survival rates for patients with small HCC (<2 cm) when this combination treatment is applied [60,61].

Combination of transarterial chemoembolization and radiofrequency ablation

Radiofrequency ablation is inherently limited in the volume of tumor that it can treat with local failure rates rising rapidly as the tumor diameter exceeds 3 cm. In animal experiments and clinical studies, TACE is shown to have synergistic effect with thermal ablation by decreasing the regional blood flow (decreased perfusion-mediated tissue cooling) and subsequently the cytotoxic effects of the chemotherapeutic drugs [62,63,64]. The combination treatment increases the zone of thermal ablation, particularly in early-stage HCC [65].

Conclusion

Curative treatments such as surgical resection, liver transplantation, and percutaneous ablation are feasible only in selected patients with early-stage HCC.

TACE is a well-established procedure, especially for patients with unresectable and intermediate to advanced HCC. RCTs and non-randomized trials have shown modest survival benefit from TACE compared to non-active treatment in such patients. Patients with well-preserved liver function (CTP Class A) and multinodular asymptomatic HCC without vascular invasion are ideal candidates for TACE. In routine practice, TACE is often used as a palliative treatment option for unresectable and advanced-stage HCC. Significant variations in TACE techniques exist with regard to: 1) choice of chemotherapeutic drug(s) (single vs. combination); 2) embolic agents (temporary agent such as gelfoam vs. permanent agents such as PVA); 3) level (segmental vs. lobar) and extent (complete vs. partial) of hepatic artery embolization; and 4) retreatment schedule. Continued technological advances and standardization of the procedure may help overcome these variations.

The current trend in locoregional treatment of HCC has been the development of multimodality treatment regimens. Combining TACE with regional ablative treatments and other techniques (radiation therapy, systemic chemotherapy, and molecular targeted therapy) may have a synergistic effect in promoting local tumor control. However, the benefit of these combination treatment strategies on overall disease recurrence and survival has not convincingly been established. There is future need for RCTs to determine the benefits of combination therapies for HCC.

REFERENCES

1. Parkin DM, Bray F, Ferlay J, and Pisani P. Estimating the world cancer burden. Globocan 2000. *Int J Cancer* 2001; **94**(2): 153–6.
2. Bosch FX, Ribes J, Diaz M, and Cleries R. Primary liver cancer: Worldwide incidence and trends. *Gastroenterology* 2004; **127**(5 Suppl 1): S5–16.
3. Okuda K, Obata H, Nakajima Y, Ohtsuki T, Okazaki N, and Ohnishi K. Prognosis of primary hepatocellular-carcinoma. *Hepatology* 1984; **4**(1 Suppl 1): S3–6.
4. Ulmer SC. Hepatocellular carcinoma: A concise guide to its status and management. *Postgrad Med* 2000; **107**(5): 117–24.
5. Llovet JM, Burroughs A, and Bruix J. Hepatocellular carcinoma. *Lancet* 2003; **362**(9399): 1907–17.
6. Yamamoto J, Okada S, Shimada K, *et al.* Treatment strategy for small hepatocellular carcinoma: Comparison of long-term results after percutaneous ethanol injection therapy and surgical resection. *Hepatology* 2001; **34**(4 Pt 1): 707–13.
7. Llovet JM, Fuster J, and Bruix J. Intention-to-treat analysis of surgical treatment for early hepatocellular carcinoma: Resection versus transplantation. *Hepatology* 1999; **30**(6): 1434–40.
8. Liu CL and Fan ST. Nonresectional therapies for hepatocellular carcinoma. *Am J Surg* 1997; **173**(4): 358–65.

9. Llovet JM and Bruix J. Systematic review of randomized trials for unresectable hepatocellular carcinoma: Chemoembolization improves survival. *Hepatology* 2003; **37**(2): 429–42.

10. Lo CM, Ngan H, Tso WK, *et al.* Randomized controlled trial of transarterial lipiodol chemoembolization for unresectable hepatocellular carcinoma. *Hepatology* 2002; **35**(5): 1164–71.

11. Okamura J, Kawai S, Ogawa M, *et al.* Prospective and randomized clinical trial for the treatment of hepatocellular carcinoma – a comparison of L-TAE with Farmorubicin and L-TAE with Adriamycin (second cooperative study). The Cooperative Study Group for Liver Cancer Treatment of Japan. *Cancer Chemother Pharmacol* 1992; **31**(Suppl): S20–4.

12. Hatanaka Y, Yamashita Y, Takahashi M, *et al.* Unresectable hepatocellular carcinoma: Analysis of prognostic factors in transcatheter management. *Radiology* 1995; **195**(3): 747–52.

13. Bismuth H. Surgical anatomy and anatomical surgery of the liver. *World J Surg* 1982; **6**(1): 3–9.

14. Hiatt JR, Gabbay J, and Busuttil RW. Surgical anatomy of the hepatic arteries in 1000 cases. *Ann Surg* 1994; **220**(1): 50–2.

15. Michels NA. Newer anatomy of liver and its variant blood supply and collateral circulation. *Am J Surg* 1966; **112**(3): 337–47.

16. Nakashima T and Kojiro M. Pathologic characteristics of hepatocellular carcinoma. *Semin Liver Dis* 1986; **6**(3): 259–66.

17. Konno T. Targeting cancer chemotherapeutic agents by use of lipiodol contrast medium. *Cancer* 1990; **66**(9): 1897–903.

18. Egawa H, Maki A, Mori K, *et al.* Effects of intra-arterial chemotherapy with a new lipophilic anticancer agent, estradiol-chlorambucil (KM2210), dissolved in lipiodol on experimental liver tumor in rats. *J Surg Oncol* 1990; **44**(2): 109–14.

19. Kruskal JB, Hlatky L, Hahnfeldt P, Teramoto K, Stokes KR, and CLouse ME. In vivo and in vitro analysis of the effectiveness of doxorubicin combined with temporary arterial occlusion in liver tumors. *J Vasc Interv Radiol* 1993; **4**(6): 741–8.

20. Nakamura H, Hashimoto T, Oi H, and Sawada S. Transcatheter oily chemoembolization of hepatocellular carcinoma. *Radiology* 1989; **170**(3 Pt 1): 783–6.

21. Llado L, Virgili J, Figueras J, *et al.* A prognostic index of the survival of patients with unresectable hepatocellular carcinoma after transcatheter arterial chemoembolization. *Cancer* 2000; **88**(1): 50–7.

22. Vogl TJ, Trapp M, Schroeder H, *et al.* Transarterial chemoembolization for hepatocellular carcinoma: Volumetric and morphologic CT criteria for assessment of prognosis and therapeutic success. Results from a liver transplantation center. *Radiology* 2000; **214**(2): 349–57.

23. Poyanli A, Rozanes I, Acunas B, and Sencer S. Palliative treatment of hepatocellular carcinoma by chemoembolization. *Acta Radiol* 2001; **42**(6): 602–7.

24. Poon RTP, Ngan H, Lo CM, Liu CL, Fan ST, and Wong J. Transarterial chemoembolization for inoperable hepatocellular carcinoma and postresection intrahepatic recurrence. *J Surg Oncol* 2000; **73**(2): 109–14.

25. Tazawa J, Maeda M, Sakai Y, *et al.* Radiation therapy in combination with transcatheter arterial chemoembolization for hepatocellular carcinoma with extensive portal vein involvement. *J Gastroenterol Hepatol* 2001; **16**(6): 660–5.

26. Gates J, Hartnell GG, Stuart KE, and Clouse ME. Chemoembolization of hepatic neoplasms: Safety, complications, and when to worry. *Radiographics* 1999; **19**(2): 399–414.

27. Kim HK, Chung YH, Song BC, *et al.* Ischemic bile duct injury as a serious complication after transarterial chemoembolization in patients with hepatocellular carcinoma. *J Clin Gastroenterol* 2001; **32**(5): 423–7.

28. Song SY, Chung JW, Han JK, *et al.* Liver abscess after transcatheter oily chemoembolization for hepatic tumors: Incidence, predisposing factors, and clinical outcome. *J Vasc Interv Radiol* 2001; **12**(3): 313–20.

29. Hirai T, Korogi Y, Ono K, *et al.* Intraarterial chemotherapy or chemoembolization for locally advanced and/or recurrent hepatic tumors: Evaluation of the feeding artery with an interventional CT system. *Cardiovasc Interv Radiol* 2001; **24**(3): 176–9.

30. Chen MS, Li JQ, Zhang YQ, *et al.* High-dose iodized oil transcatheter arterial chemoembolization for patients with large hepatocellular carcinoma. *World J Gastroenterol* 2002 Feb; **8**(1): 74–8.

31. Geschwind JF, Ramsey DE, Cleffken B, *et al.* Transcatheter arterial chemoembolization of liver tumors: Effects of embolization protocol on injectable volume of chemotherapy and subsequent arterial patency. *Cardiovasc Interv Radiol* 2003; **26**(2): 111–17.

32. Llovet JM, Real MI, Montana X, *et al.* Arterial embolisation or chemoembolisation versus symptomatic treatment in patients with unresectable hepatocellular carcinoma: A randomised controlled trial. *Lancet (North American Edition)* 2002; **359**(9319): 1734–9.

33. Lewis AL, Gonzalez MV, Lloyd AW, *et al.* DC bead: In vitro characterization of a drug-delivery device for transarterial chemoembolization. *J Vasc Interv Radiol* 2006; **17**(2): 335–42.

34. Malagari K, Chatzimichael K, Alexopoulou E, *et al.* Transarterial chemoembolization of unresectable hepatocellular carcinoma with drug eluting beads: Results of an open-label study of 62 patients. Clinical report. *Cardiovasc Interv Radiol* 2008; **31**(2): 269–80.

35. Kettenbach J, Stadler A, Katzler IV, *et al.* Drug-loaded microspheres for the treatment of liver cancer: Review of current results. *Cardiovasc Interv Radiol* 2008; **31**(3): 468–76.

36. Wigmore SJ, Redhead DN, Thomson BN, *et al.* Postchemoembolisation syndrome – tumour necrosis or hepatocyte injury? *Br J Cancer* 2003; **89**(8): 1423–7.

37. Sakamoto I, Aso N, Nagaoki K, *et al.* Complications associated with transcatheter arterial embolization for hepatic tumors. *Radiographics* 1998; **18**(3): 605–19.

38. Chung J, Park JH, Han JK, *et al.* Hepatic tumors: Predisposing factors for complications of transcatheter oily chemoembolization. *Radiology* 1996; **198**(1): 33–40.

39. Chung JW, Park JH, Im JG, Han JK, and Han MC. Pulmonary oil embolism after transcatheter oily chemoembolization of hepatocellular carcinoma. *Radiology* 1993; **187**(3): 689–93.

40. Huo TI, Wu JC, Lee PC, Chang FY, and Lee SD. Incidence and risk factors for acute renal failure in patients with hepatocellular carcinoma undergoing transarterial chemoembolization: A prospective study. *Liver Int* 2004; **24**(3): 210–15.

41. Savastano S, Miotto D, Casarrubea G, Teso S, Chiesura-Corona M, and Feltrin GP. Transcatheter arterial chemoembolization for hepatocellular carcinoma in patients with Child's grade A or B cirrhosis: A multivariate analysis of prognostic factors. *J Clin Gastroenterol* 1999; **28**(4): 334–40.

42. Ahn SH, Han KH, Park JY, *et al.* Treatment outcome of transcatheter arterial chemoinfusion according to anticancer agents and prognostic factors in patients with advanced hepatocellular carcinoma (TNM stage IVa). *Yonsei Med J* 2004; **45**(5): 847–58.

43. Kiely J, Rilling WS, Touzios JG, *et al.* Chemoembolization in patients at high risk: Results and complications. *J Vasc Interv Radiol* 2006; **17**(1): 47–53.

44. Kothary N, Weintraub JL, Susman J, and Rundback JH. Transarterial chemoembolization for primary hepatocellular carcinoma in patients at high risk. *J Vasc Interv Radiol* 2007; **18**(12): 1517–26.

45. Camma C, Schepis F, Orlando A, *et al.* Transarterial chemoembolization for unresectable hepatocellular carcinoma: Meta-analysis of randomized controlled trials. *Radiology* 2002; **224**(1): 47–54.

46. Takayasu K, Shima Y, Muramatsu Y, *et al.* Hepatocellular carcinoma treatment with intraarterial iodized oil with and without chemotherapeutic-agents. *Radiology* 1987; **163**(2): 345–51.

47. Matsui O, Kadoya M, Yoshikawa J, Gabata T, Takashima T, and Demachi H. Subsegmental transcatheter arterial embolization for small hepatocellular carcinomas: Local therapeutic effect and 5-year survival rate. *Cancer Chemother Pharmacol* 1994; **33**(Suppl): S84–8.

48. Ramsey WH and Wu GY. Hepatocellular carcinoma: Update on diagnosis and treatment. *Dig Dis* 1995; **13**(2): 81–91.

49. Spreafico C, Marchiano A, Regalia E, *et al.* Chemoembolization of hepatocellular carcinoma in patients who undergo liver transplantation. *Radiology* 1994; **192**(3): 687–90.

50. Stefanini GF, Amorati P, Biselli M, *et al.* Efficacy of transarterial targeted treatments on survival of patients with hepatocellular carcinoma: An Italian experience. *Cancer* 1995; **75**(10): 2427–34.

51. Rose AT, Rose DM, Pinson CW, *et al.* Hepatocellular carcinoma outcomes based on indicated treatment strategy. *Am Surg* 1998; **64**(12): 1128–34.

52. Bismuth H, Morino M, Sherlock D, *et al.* Primary treatment of hepatocellular carcinoma by arterial chemoembolization. *Am J Surg* 1992; **163**(4): 387–94.

53. Matsui O, Kadoya M, Yoshikawa J, Gabata T, Takashima T, and Demachi H. Subsegmental transcatheter arterial embolization for small hepatocellular carcinomas: Local therapeutic effect and 5-year survival rate. *Cancer Chemother Pharmacol* 1994; **33**(Suppl): S84–8.

54. Vetter D, Wenger JJ, Bergier JM, Doffoel M, and Bockel R. Transcatheter oily chemoembolization in the management of advanced hepatocellular carcinoma in cirrhosis: Results of a western comparative study in 60 patients. *Hepatology* 1991; **13**(3): 427–33.

55. Zhang Z, Liu Q, He J, Yang J, Yang G, and Wu M. The effect of preoperative transcatheter hepatic arterial chemoembolization on disease-free survival after hepatectomy for hepatocellular carcinoma. *Cancer* 2000; **89**(12): 2606–12.

56. Richard HM III, Silberzweig JE, Mitty HA, Lou WY, Ahn J, and Cooper JM. Hepatic arterial complications in liver transplant recipients treated with pretransplantation chemoembolization for hepatocellular carcinoma. *Radiology* 2000; **214**(3): 775–9.

57. Veltri A, Grosso M, Martina MC, *et al.* Effect of preoperative radiological treatment of hepatocellular carcinoma before liver transplantation: A retrospective study. *Cardiovasc Interv Radiol* 1998; **21**(5): 393–8.

58. Decaens T, Roudot-Thoraval F, Bresson-Hadni S, *et al.* Impact of pretransplantation transarterial chemoembolization on survival and recurrence after liver transplantation for hepatocellular carcinoma. *Liver Transplant* 2005; **11**(7): 767–75.

59. Chan ES, Chow PK, Tai B, Machin D, and Soo K. Neoadjuvant and adjuvant therapy for operable hepatocellular carcinoma. *Cochrane Database of Systematic Reviews.* 2000(2):CD001199.

60. Bartolozzi C, Lencioni R, Caramella D, *et al.* Treatment of large HCC: Transcatheter arterial chemoembolization combined with percutaneous ethanol injection versus repeated transcatheter arterial chemoembolization. *Radiology* 1995; **197**(3): 812–18.

61. Kamada K, Kitamoto M, Aikata H, *et al.* Combination of transcatheter arterial chemoembolization using cisplatin-lipiodol suspension and percutaneous ethanol injection for treatment of advanced small hepatocellular carcinoma. *Am J Surg* 2002; **184**(3): 284–90.

62. Ahmed M, Lukyanov AN, Torchilin V, Tournier H, Schneider AN, and Goldberg SN. Combined radiofrequency ablation and adjuvant liposomal chemotherapy: Effect of chemotherapeutic agent, nanoparticle size, and circulation time. *J Vasc Interv Radiol* 2005; **16**(10): 1365–71.

63. Rossi S, Garbagnati F, Lencioni R, *et al.* Percutaneous radio-frequency thermal ablation of nonresectable hepatocellular carcinoma after occlusion of tumor blood supply. *Radiology* 2000; **217**(1): 119–26.

64. Higgins M, Mondschein J, and Stavropoulos S. Combined chemoembolization and percutaneous radiofrequency ablation for local control of liver tumors. *J Vasc Interv Radiol* 2007; **18**(2): S46–7.

65. Yamakado K, Nakatsuka A, Takaki H, *et al.* Early-stage hepatocellular carcinoma: Radiofrequency ablation combined with chemoembolization versus hepatectomy. *Radiology* 2008; **247**(1): 260–6.

b. Ablation of hepatocellular carcinoma

Elaine M. Caoili

History

The standard treatment of hepatocellular carcinoma (HCC) consists of hepatectomy or liver transplantation; however, not all patients are surgical candidates due to a number of factors such as poor liver function, advanced disease, or other medical comorbidities. Due to the persistent need for alternative therapies, there has been increased interest in minimally invasive, image-guided ablative therapies, particularly radiofrequency ablation (RFA).

The basic concept of using radiofrequency waves to create thermal energy was first described in 1891 by D'Arsonval, who found that, as radiofrequency waves were passed through tissues, temperatures rose [1]. However, it was only after 1928, with the introduction of the Bovie knife, that the use of radiofrequency waves became more common in medical applications [2]. In 1990, McGahan *et al.* [3] and Rossi *et al.* [4] independently modified the technology of the Bovie knife and found that, by using radiofrequency currents, a percutaneously placed insulated needle could create an area of focal necrosis in the tissues surrounding the needle. Since then, variations of radiofrequency generators and needles have been developed for the use of ablative therapy. Technical advances in generators have increased the amount of power that can be deposited into a targeted region increasing the amount of tissue necrosis. Improvements in needle designs (multiprobe arrays vs. internally cooled electrodes) have increased the potential volume of treated tumor. Even now, new strategies are being developed to increase the amount of tissue necrosis created by RFA, both alone or in combination with other therapies, thereby increasing the applications and continued use of this technique for the treatment of tumors in the future.

Primary Carcinomas of the Liver, ed. Hero K. Hussain and Isaac R. Francis. Published by Cambridge University Press. © Cambridge University Press 2010.

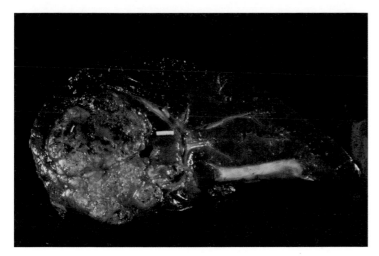

Figure 3.1 HCC (*white line*) in a non-cirrhotic liver. Tumor varies from firm and pale to necrotic and hemorrhagic.

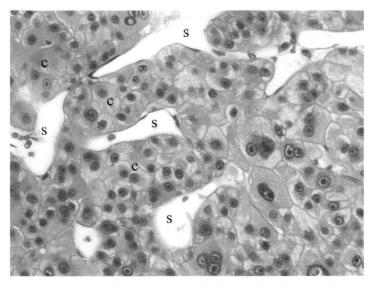

Figure 3.2 The trabecular pattern of HCC is characterized by cords of neoplastic hepatocytes (c) separated by sinusoid-like vascular spaces (s). The neoplasms differ from benign liver cells in having cells with increased ratios of nuclear-to-cytoplasmic volumes and enlarged nuclei with macronucleoli, and by having broader trabeculae. (hematoxylin and eosin [H&E], ×200)

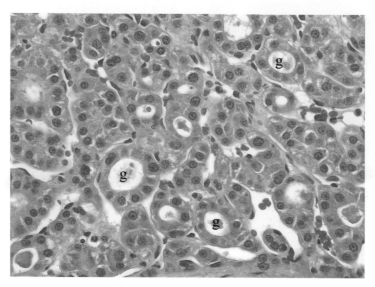

Figure 3.3 The pseudoglandular pattern of HCC has glandlike spaces that are dilated bile canaliculi between neoplastic hepatocytes (g). Many of these spaces contain inspissated bile. (H&E, ×200)

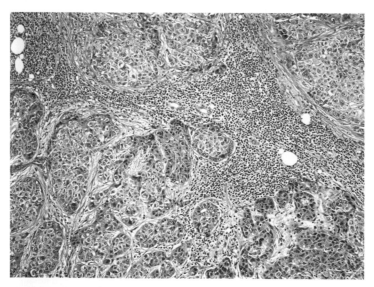

Figure 3.4 In scirrhous HCC, nests of tumor cells are separated by fibrous stroma, often containing a prominent lymphocytic infiltrate. (H&E, ×100)

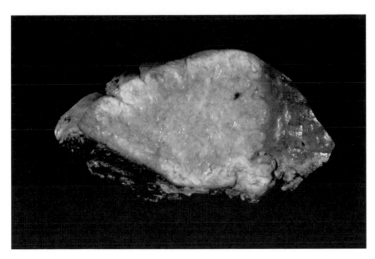

Figure 3.5 This fibrolamellar variant of HCC is present immediately beneath the capsular surface. The tumor is paler than the adjacent red-brown normal parenchyma, and has multiple, white fibrous bands that traverse the mass.

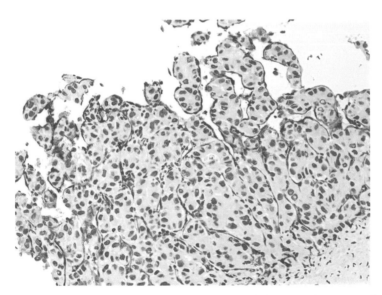

Figure 3.6 The endothelial cells lining the sinusoid-like spaces in HCC are often immunohistochemically positive with antibodies to CD34 (*brown stain* along the edges of tumor cells), unlike normal liver, which lacks such CD34 expression along sinusoids. (CD34 immunohistochemical stain, ×200)

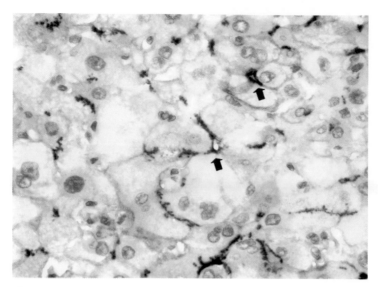

Figure 3.7 Bile canalicular immunohistochemical positivity with CD10 (*arrows*) is a feature of both benign and neoplastic liver, and can be used as evidence of hepatocellular differentiation. (CD10 immunohistochemical stain, ×400)

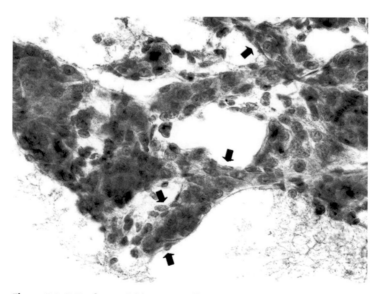

Figure 3.8 FNA of HCC yields tumor cells arranged in anastomosing cords, partially covered by endothelial cells (*arrows*). The cells have larger nuclei, less cytoplasm, and are more crowded than normal hepatocytes. (Papanicolaou stain, ×200)

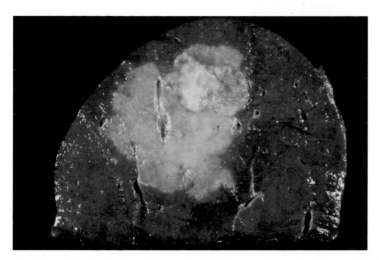

Figure 3.9 This cholangiocarcinoma is a single, non-encapsulated mass. It is dense and nearly white due to the abundant fibrous stroma that is typical of cholangiocarcinoma.

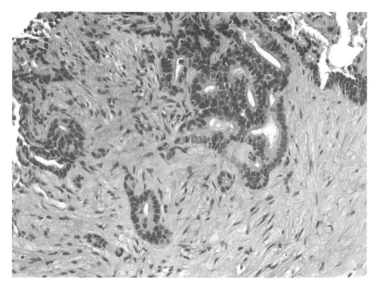

Figure 3.10 Most cholangiocarcinomas are composed of well-formed neoplastic tubules present within abundant fibrous stroma. (H&E, ×100)

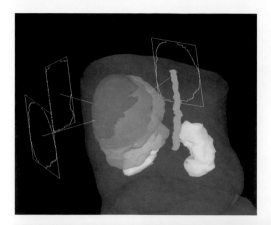

Figure 7.2a.1 Example of beam arrangement and field shapes used to treat a large HCC. The liver is shown in *gray,* PTV in *red,* kidneys in *yellow,* and spinal cord in *green.*

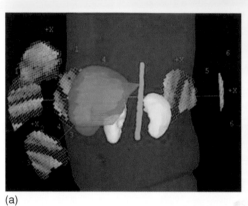

(a)

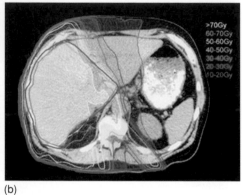

(b)

Figure 7.2a.2 IMRT treatment for a patient with unresectable HCC. (a): Solid-surface reconstruction of the PTV (*red*), liver (*purple*), right and left kidneys (*yellow*), and the spinal cord (*green*) are shown, along with the projections of six IMRT fields, with the dose intensity in each beamlet represented by gray-scale. (b): Distribution of dose at the level of central axis.

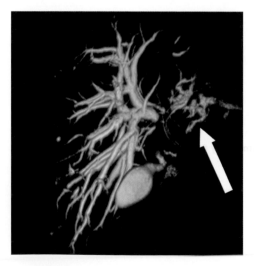

Figure 9.10 Volume-rendered MRCP image showing crowding of the left hepatic ducts (*arrow*) secondary to atrophy of the left lobe. The atrophy was secondary to obstruction of the left duct and left portal vein by a cholangiocarcinoma extending predominantly into the left lobe.

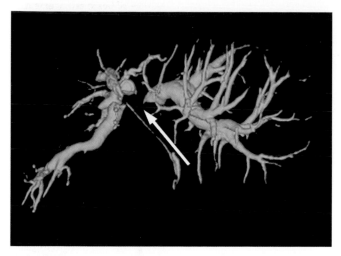

Figure 10.2b Intraductal cholangiocarcinoma (*arrows*) at the ductal bifurcation confirmed at surgery. The tumor is seen as signal loss on the volume-rendered MRCP image (b). The latter is generated from the three-dimensional MRCP series.

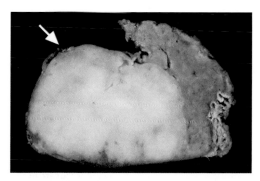

Figure 12.3f Lipid rich-AML (*arrow*) mimicking a lipoma in segment VII of the liver. (f): Gross histopathologic specimen photograph demonstrates the lesion (*arrow*). Initial biopsies performed at an outside hospital revealed a diagnosis of hepatic lipoma. Because of persistent right upper quadrant discomfort and the patient's desire for surgical management, the lesion was removed via laparoscopy. Although the macroscopic features suggest a predominantly fat-containing lesion, immunohistochemical staining was positive for HMB-45, leading to a diagnosis of a lipid-rich AML.

Mechanism of destruction

During RFA, a closed-loop circuit is created by placing a patient, a needle electrode, a generator, and dispersive electrodes (grounding pads) in series. A high-frequency alternating electric current (200–1200 kHz) passes from the active electrode into the patient's tissue. The tissue ions attempt to follow the changes in the direction of the current, but because the tissues are resistant to the current in comparison to the electrodes, the ions in the tissues surrounding the electrodes are agitated. The ionic agitation is converted to heat by means of friction. The current associated with the grounding pads is dispersed over a larger surface area, unlike that associated with the needle electrode. Thus, the heat generated by the needle electrode is intense and focused to the tissues surrounding it. This heat can cause irreversible tissue damage leading to cellular necrosis [5,6].

Cellular necrosis or coagulative necrosis is dependent on the tissue temperature achieved and the duration of the heating. Irreparable cellular damage occurs when temperatures reach 50–55°C for 4 to 6 minutes. Further damage to mitochondrial and cytosolic enzymes occurs between 60 and 100°C, and this damage leads to nearly immediate coagulation of tissues. At 100°C or greater, tissue vaporizes and carbonizes. This produces tissue charring and gas, which increase the resistance of the tissues, preventing heat conduction. Thus, a goal of RFA for tumor destruction is to achieve temperatures of 50–100°C in the entire targeted volume for 10 to 30 minutes, given the slow conduction of thermal energy from the needle electrode through the tissues [5,6].

In an effort to better understand the technical factors that affect ablation zone size, investigators such as Goldberg *et al.* [7] focused on the effects of electrode size, tip temperature, and treatment duration in ex vivo liver and muscle. Goldberg *et al.* showed that the size of the zone or cavity correlated with the diameter of the electrode and the duration of the RF application. These investigators also demonstrated that the length of the zone correlated with the length of the uninsulated portion of the needle electrode. Similar results were found in vivo [8]; however, the cavity diameters achieved were smaller, and higher temperatures were required to achieve coagulative necrosis. It was postulated that perfusion-mediated tissue cooling likely explained the decreased effectiveness in vivo. To increase the diameter of the ablation cavity, Goldberg *et al.* evaluated the effect of using several needle electrodes while varying configuration and spacing. Simultaneous application of the electrodes resulted in a larger volume of necrosis in comparison to sequential application of the electrodes. Also, spacing of the electrodes greater than 1.5 cm apart resulted in unaffected areas of tissue between areas of necrosis [9].

Improving technology/techniques

Effective ablative therapy is dependent on achieving and maintaining sufficient heat production and minimizing heat loss. Heat production is dependent on the equipment used as well as the tissue being heated. Heterogeneity in tissue such as fibrosis, fat, or fluid will alter electrical and thermal conductance. Heat is mainly lost through vascular circulation via nearby blood vessels, but heat loss also occurs at increasing distances from the electrode limiting the zone of coagulation. Thus, there are several factors that can limit the zone of coagulation, and this has led investigators to develop strategies to improve RFA.

In an effort to increase the heating efficacy of ablation therapy, manufacturers increased the wattage of commercially available generators in order to increase the amount of current deposited in the tissues. Another modification consisted of generators that alternated high-frequency energy currents with minimal currents for defined time periods in order to achieve better current deposition in tissues. This modification provided tissue cooling adjacent to the electrode without affecting the heating in deeper tissues allowing for greater energy deposition and tissue coagulation [10]. In addition, in order to facilitate the ablative treatment, manufacturers developed commercially available systems that monitor the ablation process (RITA Medical Systems, Radionics, and RadioTherapeutics). These systems can evaluate tissue temperature or tissue impedance and can automatically reduce generator current output when tissue temperatures reach or exceed a target temperature or when tissue impedance increases. Electrodes were also modified with designs such as the multiprobe array system (Starburst XL and Starburst Xli; RITA Medical Systems; Leveen Needle Electrode; RadioTherapeutics) in order to deposit thermal energy within a larger volume of tissue. The multiprobe array consists of a large (typically 14-gauge) insulated cannula containing a number of retractable, curved wires that can be manually advanced in a preset configuration ensuring adequate distances between the wires. Another development was the use of an internally cooled electrode designed to prevent excessive tissue heating. Within the electrode is an internal channel though which chilled fluid is circulated during the ablation. The cooling prevents tissue charring adjacent to the needle and allows increased generator output. This leads to increased volumes of coagulation necrosis [11,12].

Several investigators have found that saline injection into the tumor increases coagulation volume by improving tissue heat conduction [13,14,15]. Tissue electrical conductivity is altered by injecting saline prior to or during ablation. Saline increases tissue ionicity allowing for greater energy deposition; however, results are unpredictable and in fact saline can increase the energy requirements for cellular death [16]. Other investigations have focused on decreasing perfusion-mediated cooling of the ablation zone. Experiments in which hepatic blood flow is altered demonstrated that vascular occlusion enhances the size of the thermal ablation. Strategies to decrease blood flow during ablation have included angiographic balloon occlusion of the hepatic artery, which has been found useful for hypervascular tumors [17]. Another strategy includes portal venous and hepatic artery occlusion (Pringle maneuver) at surgery. Clinical results using the Pringle maneuver have been reported to be promising [18,19], allowing for treatment of larger tumors. Pharmacologic modulation of blood flow has also been evaluated but is still considered experimental [20].

The role of imaging

Imaging plays a critical role in percutaneous RFA by 1) determining the number, size, and location of tumors and 2) providing guidance for accurate and safe needle placement. Computed tomography (CT) and magnetic resonance imaging (MRI) are used to determine if patients are eligible for RFA. Ideally, tumor should be confined to the liver without evidence of metastatic disease or vascular invasion. The tumor should be less than 4 to 5 cm in diameter, with a maximum of four to five lesions. Ultrasound and CT have been commonly used to guide RFA. Ultrasound provides convenient real-time visualization, is low cost, and is widely available. CT allows visualization of all organs and soft tissues including those containing bone or air. Each modality has its advantages and disadvantages, and which is chosen to provide guidance is often operator dependent. At our center, we prefer to use ultrasound for RFA and use CT only in rare instances when access or tumor visibility is poor with ultrasound. The imaging used should clearly depict the targeted tumor as well as a safe pathway for the needle electrode(s) in order to prevent nearby organ injury (Figure 7.1b.1a). Liver tumors should be approached using the most direct path without traversing hepatic vessels or other organs such as the gallbladder, colon, diaphragm, and lung. Also, a path traversing normal hepatic parenchyma prior to reaching the tumor is recommended in order to prevent extracapsular bleeding or tract seeding (Figure 7.1b.1b).

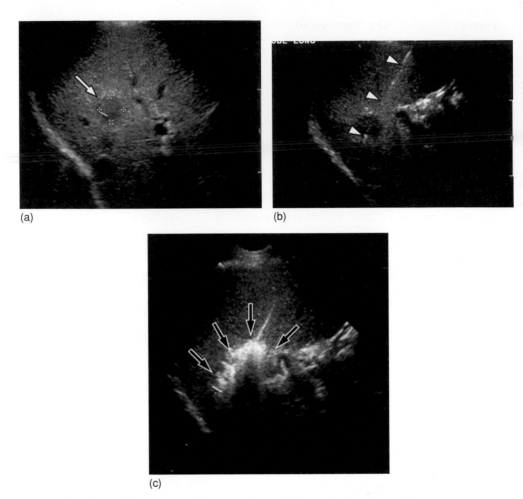

(a)   (b)

(c)

Figure 7.1b.1 (a–c): Fifty-one-year-old man with hepatitis C complicated with HCC, status postresection. Ultrasound image demonstrates a 1.3-cm recurrent tumor in the right hepatic lobe (*arrow*) (a). Under real imaging guidance, a needle electrode (*arrowheads*) is placed into a small HCC (b). Ablated tissue appears hyperechoic (*black arrows*) during ultrasound monitoring due to the creation of gas within the cavity (c).

Electrodes should be carefully placed as multiple punctures may lead to tumor spillage. The needle electrodes must be visualized so that adjustments in needle positioning can be easily performed in order to ensure that the active tip of the electrode is located within the tumor. Large tumors may require placement of several electrodes to perform overlapping ablations in order to treat the tumor as well as a 5- to 10-mm margin of normal tissue. During ablation therapy, the ablated tissues appear hyperechoic at ultrasound monitoring due to the formation of gas

(Figure 7.1b.1c). On unenhanced and enhanced CT, the area appears as a well-demarcated region of hypodensity often containing foci of gas. On pathologic examination, CT was found to better depict the volume of ablated liver tissue in comparison to ultrasound [21].

Follow-up imaging is crucial to 1) assess treatment efficacy and 2) evaluate for recurrent tumor. At our institution, follow-up imaging is typically performed with contrast-enhanced MRI; however, it can be performed with either contrast-enhanced CT or MRI. On initial postablation imaging, a successful ablation is indicated by a cavity corresponding to the location of the initial tumor and one which is larger in size than the original tumor, due to inclusion of the tumor and safety margins. However, when treating HCC in the cirrhotic liver, the ablation cavity tends to be similar in size to the original tumor, as the radiofrequency current does not pass easily out of the tumor due to the increased impedance of cirrhotic hepatic parenchyma [22,23,24]. The ablation cavity appears as a well-defined, round or oval, non-enhancing region on contrast-enhanced CT or MRI. Foci of higher attenuation can be found within the cavity corresponding to coagulation necrosis, especially on unenhanced CT images. On unenhanced T1-weighted images, the ablation cavity is often hyperintense. On T2-weighted images, the treated area is hypointense, but foci of high signal intensity within the cavity can be seen. Contrast-enhanced T1-weighted images demonstrate a hypointense region that may have a thin rim of enhancement. The cavity will eventually decrease in size within 12 months of the ablation. A study of 43 HCCs treated with RFA showed a decrease in volume of 21% at 1 month, 50% at 4 months, 65% at 7 months, and 89% at 16 months [25]. Wedge-shaped areas of contrast enhancement can be seen on arterial-phase imaging and are thought to be due to perfusion anomalies such as arterioportal fistulas [25]. Also, a thin (2 mm) peripheral rim of enhancement surrounding the cavity is often more apparent during the equilibrium phase of imaging and is thought to be due to inflammatory tissue with neovascularization [25,26] (Figure 7.1b.2a–c). With time, this rim becomes less conspicuous [25,27]. This rim was identified in 24% and 18% of ablated tumors on MRI and CT, respectively, at 2 months and in 2% on MRI at 9-month follow-up [25]. Residual tumor typically presents as arterially enhancing nodules or irregular thickening at the periphery of the ablation cavity (Figure 7.1b.3a–c) in the majority of cases; however, recurrence can also occur remote from the ablation site. Also, an increase in cavity size suggests incomplete treatment [28]. It has been demonstrated that local recurrent tumors will typically present within 12 months of the ablative therapy [25,29].

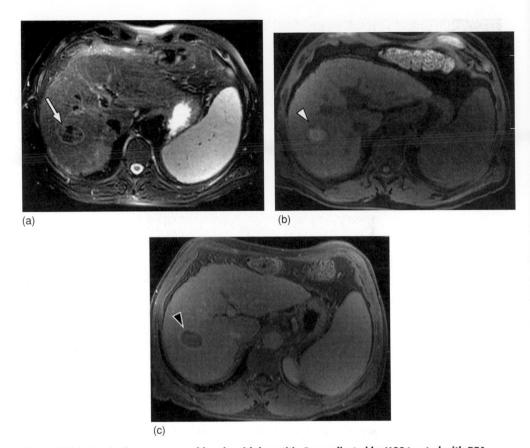

(a)   (b)

(c)

Figure 7.1b.2 (a–c): Sixty-one-year-old male with hepatitis C complicated by HCC treated with RFA. Three-month MRI follow-up demonstrates successful treatment without recurrence. T2-weighted image shows central hypointensity within the cavity with a peripheral hyperintense rim (*arrow*) (a). T1-weighted image shows central hyperintensity within the cavity with a peripheral hypointense rim (*arrowhead*) (b). Contrast-enhanced T1-weighted image shows no enhancement within the cavity with thin rim enhancement (*black arrowhead*), consistent with inflammation or fibrosis (c).

Complications

The complication rate of percutaneous RFA therapy ranges from 2 to 36% with a mortality rate of 0–2% [30,31,32,33]. Complications related to needle electrode placement are bleeding, infection, and tumor seeding. Complications can also be related to thermal energy damage to nearby structures resulting in bowel perforation and grounding pad skin burns. Vascular complications such as pseudoaneurysm, arteriovenous fistula, hepatic and portal vein thrombosis, and hepatic venous infarction have been reported. Postablation abscess typically develops 2 to 8 weeks after ablation and may require catheter drainage as well as antibiotic therapy.

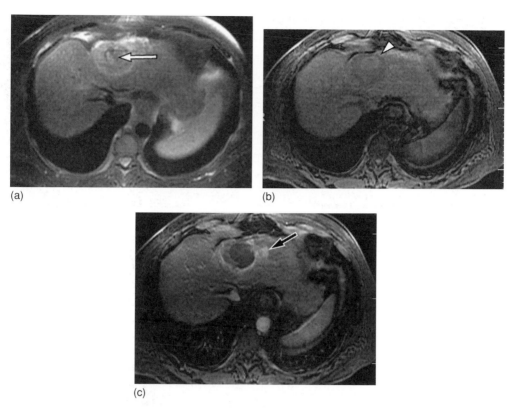

(a)

(b)

(c)

Figure 7.1b.3 (a–c): Fifty-three-year-old male with hepatitis C complicated by HCC treated with RFA. One-month MRI follow-up demonstrates residual tumor. T2-weighted image shows central hyperintensity within the cavity (*arrow*) (a). T1-weighted image shows central hyperintensity within the cavity surrounded by a thick rim of hypointensity (*arrowhead*) (b). Contrast-enhanced T1-weighted image shows a posterior, medial thick nodular rim of arterial enhancement, consistent with residual tumor (*black arrow*) (c).

Tumor seeding has been seen 3 to 12 months after ablation and is more likely to occur with aggressive tumors and/or subcapsular location and in patients with high levels of alpha-fetoprotein [34]. Minor complications such as pain, fever, nausea, and loose stools are common. A postablation syndrome consisting of flu-like symptoms and low-grade fevers may be seen in cases involving large tumor (>4 cm) ablations. The symptoms are self-limiting, usually resolve within 10 days, and require supportive therapy of rest and pain medication [32,35].

Efficacy: Survival rates

Several studies have focused on the use of RFA in treating HCC; however, most of these investigations are patient series or non-randomized trials. Large clinical series have shown that the 5-year survival rates post-RFA vary between 33 and 55%, which is comparable to survival rates after hepatic resection [36,37,38,39]. For example, in a prospective study by Montorsi *et al.* [40], the investigators treated patients with Child–Turcotte–Pugh Class A or B cirrhosis and a single HCC (<5 cm) with laparoscopic RFA or surgery and found the 4-year survival rates to be similar for both groups of patients; however, RFA did result in significantly higher recurrence rates. In another study, Raut *et al.* [41] compared percutaneous RFA, open surgical RFA, and open surgical RFA with hepatic resection in 194 patients with HCC. Early survival was worse for those patients who underwent resection and RFA likely due to the increased morbidity associated with resection; however, there was no significant difference in the 5-year survival rates among the three groups. In one randomized controlled trial by Chen *et al.* [42], similar results were also found. Chen *et al.* compared RFA to surgical hepatic resection and found that disease-free survival was comparable between the two treatments.

Efficacy: Intrahepatic recurrence of hepatocellular carcinoma

Unfortunately, intrahepatic recurrence of HCC after RFA is common, varying from 2 to 53% [29,41,43,44,45,46,47]. Risk factors include large tumor size [44,46,47], multiple nodules [48], and subcapsular or perivascular location [49,50]. In a retrospective analysis, Lam *et al.* [47] found that, although there was no difference in survival between patients with and without local recurrence, tumor size greater than 2.5 cm was a significant risk factor for recurrence. Interestingly, these investigators also demonstrated that late recurrence (>12 months) had a significantly better prognosis than early recurrence for overall survival rates [47].

Unfortunately, there often is a discrepancy between imaging and pathologic examination of the ablation cavity. In studies of explanted livers, zones of complete ablation seen on both CT and MRI did not always correspond with complete coagulative necrosis on pathological examination [51,52]. For example, Lu *et al.* [51], in a study of 24 post-RFA CT ($n = 23$) and MRI ($n = 1$) examinations, found the sensitivity and specificity for the detection of residual or recurrent hepatocellular carcinoma following RFA to be 36% and 100%, respectively. This fact emphasizes the importance of short-interval imaging follow-up after RFA in order to detect early recurrent tumors as well as the need for improved imaging detection.

Summary

The feasibility and safety of RFA therapy have been well documented, and the clinical efficacy of this treatment has been encouraging. Investigators are now looking into furthering the application of ablative therapies by combining them with other treatments such as chemotherapy as well as other local therapies such as transarterial chemoembolization. Thus, RFA and other minimally invasive ablative therapies continue to evolve and play an increasing role in the management and treatment of HCC.

REFERENCES

1. D'Arsonval MA. Action physiologique des courants alternatifs. *CR Soc Biol* 1891; **43**: 283–6.
2. Cushing H and Bovie WT. Electro-surgery as an aid to the removal of intracranial tumors. *Surg Gynecol Obstetr* 1928; **47**: 751–84.
3. McGahan JP, Browning PD, Brock JM, and Tesluk H. Hepatic ablation using radiofrequency electrocautery. *Invest Radiol* 1990; **25**: 267–70.
4. Rossi S, Fornari F, Pathies C, and Buscarini L. Thermal lesions induced by 480 KHz localized current field in guinea pig and pig liver. *Tumori* 1990; **76**: 54–7.
5. Rhim H, Goldberg SN, Dodd GD III, *et al.* Essential techniques for successful radiofrequency thermal ablation of malignant hepatic tumors. *Radiographics* 2001; **21**: S17–35.
6. Gazelle GS, Goldberg SN, Solbiati L, and Livraghi T. Tumor ablation with radiofrequency energy. *Radiology* 2000; **217**: 633–46.
7. Goldberg SN, Gazelle GS, Dawson SL, Rittman WJ, Mueller PR, and Rosenthal DI. Tissue ablation with radiofrequency: Effect of probe size, gauge, duration and temperature on lesion volume. *Acad Radiol* 1995; **2**: 399–404.
8. Goldberg SN, Gazelle GS, Halpern EF, Rittman WJ, and Mueller PR. Radiofrequency tissue ablation: Importance of local temperature along the electrode tip exposure in determining lesion size and shape. *Acad Radiol* 1996; **3**: 212–18.
9. Goldberg SN, Gazelle GS, Dawson SL, Rittman WJ, Mueller PR, and Rosenthal DI. Tissue ablation with radiofrequency using multiprobe arrays. *Acad Radiol* 1995; **2**: 670–4.
10. Goldberg SN, Stein M, Gazelle GS, Kruskal JB, and Clouse ME. Percutaneous radiofrequency tissue ablation: Optimization of pulsed RF-technique to increase coagulation necrosis. *J Vasc Interv Radiol* 1999; **10**: 907–16.
11. Goldberg SN and Gazelle GS. Radiofrequency tissue ablation and techniques for increasing coagulation necrosis. *Hepato-Gastroenterology* 2001; **48**: 359–67.
12. Goldberg SN, Solbiati L, Hahn PF, *et al.* Large-volume ablation with radiofrequency by using a clustered, internally cooled electrode technique: Laboratory and clinical experience in liver metastases. *Radiology* 1998; **209**: 371–9.

13. Miao Y, Ni Y, Yu J, and Marchal G. A comparative study on validation of a novel cooled-wet electrode for radiofrequency liver ablation. *Invest Radiol* 2000; **35**: 438–44.

14. Curley MG and Hamilton PS. Creation of large thermal lesions in liver using saline-enhanced RF ablation. Proceedings of the 19th International Conference of IEEE/EMBS. 1997: 2516–19.

15. Livraghi T, Goldberg SN, Monti F, *et al.* Saline-enhanced radiofrequency tissue ablation in the treatment of liver metastases. *Radiology* 1997; **202**: 205–10.

16. Goldberg SN, Ahmed M, Gazelle GS, *et al.* Radiofrequency thermal ablation with adjuvant saline injection: Effect of electrical conductivity on tissue heating and coagulation. *Radiology* 2001; **219**: 157–65.

17. Rossi S, Garbagnati F, Lencioni R, *et al.* Percutaneous radio-frequency thermal ablation of non-resectable hepatocellular carcinoma after occlusion of tumor blood supply. *Radiology* 2000; **217**: 119–26.

18. Goldberg SN, Hahn PF, Tanabe KK, *et al.* Percutaneous radiofrequency tissue ablation: Does perfusion-mediated tissue cooling limit coagulation necrosis? *J Vasc Interv Radiol* 1998; **9**: 101–11.

19. Curley SA, Izzo F, Delrio P, *et al.* Radiofrequency ablation of unresectable primary and metastatic hepatic malignancies: Results in 123 patients. *Ann Surg* 1999; **230**: 1–8.

20. Goldberg SN, Hahn PF, Halpern E, Fogle R, and Gazelle GS. Radio-frequency tissue ablation: Effect of pharmacologic modulation of blood flow on coagulation diameter. *Radiology* 1998; **209**: 761–7.

21. Cha CH, Lee FT, Gurney JM, *et al.* CT versus sonography for monitoring radiofrequency ablation in a porcine liver. *Am J Radiol* 2000; **175**: 705–11.

22. Lencioni R, Cioni D, and Bartolozzi C. Percutaneous radiofrequency thermal ablation of liver malignancies: Techniques, indications, imaging findings, and clinical results. *Abdom Imaging* 2000; **26**: 345–60.

23. Rossi S, Di Stasi M, Buscarini E, *et al.* Percutaneous radiofrequency interstitial thermal ablation in the treatment of small hepatocellular carcinoma. *Cancer J Sci Am* 1995; **1**: 73–7.

24. Livraghi T, Goldberg SN, Lazzaroni S, *et al.* Small hepatocellular carcinoma: Treatment with radiofrequency ablation versus ethanol injection. *Radiology* 1999; **210**: 235–40.

25. Dromain C, de Baere T, Elias D, *et al.* Hepatic tumors treated with percutaneous radiofrequency ablation: CT and MR imaging follow-up. *Radiology* 2002; **223**: 255–62.

26. Goldberg SN, Gazelle GS, Compton CC, Mueller PR, and Tanabe KK. Treatment of intrahepatic malignancy with radiofrequency ablation: Radiologic-pathologic correlation. *Cancer* 2000; **88**: 2452–63.

27. Tsuda M, Majima K, Yamda T, Saitou H, Ishibashi T, and Takahashi S. Hepatocellular carcinoma after radiofrequency ablation therapy: Dynamic CT evaluation of treatment. *Clin Imaging* 2001; **25**: 409–15.

28. Chopra S, Dodd GD III, Chintapalli KN, Leyendecker JR, Karahan OI, and Rhim H. Tumor recurrence after radiofrequency thermal ablation of hepatic tumors: Spectrum of findings on dual-phase contrast-enhanced CT. *AJR Am J Roentgenol* 2001; **177**: 381–7.

29. Curley SA, Izzo F, Ellis LM, Vauthey JN, and Vallone P. Radiofrequency ablation of hepatocellular cancer in 110 patients with cirrhosis. *Ann Surg* 2000; **232**: 381–91.

30. Livraghi T, Solbiati L, Meloni MF, Gazelle GS, Halpern EF, and Goldberg SN. Treatment of focal liver tumors with percutaneous radiofrequency ablation: Complications encountered in a multicenter study. *Radiology* 2003; **226**: 441–51.

31. Rhim H, Yoon KH, Lee JM, *et al.* Major complications after radio-frequency thermal ablation of hepatic tumors: Spectrum of imaging findings. *Radiographics* 2003; **23**: 123–34.

32. Rhim H, Dodd GD III, Chintapalli KN, *et al.* Radiofrequency thermal ablation of abdominal tumors: Lesson learned from complications. *Radiographics* 2004; **24**: 41–52.

33. Akahane M, Koga H, Kato N, *et al.* Complications of percutaneous radiofrequency ablation for hepatocellular carcinoma: Imaging spectrum and management. *Radiographics* 2006; **25**: S57–68.

34. Llovet JM, Vilana R, Bru C, *et al.* Increased risk of tumor seeding after percutaneous radiofrequency ablation for single hepatocellular carcinoma. *Hepatology* 2001; **33**: 1124–9.

35. Wah TM, Arellano RS, Gervais DA, Saltalamacchia CA, Martino J, and Halpern EF. Image-guided percutaneous radiofrequency ablation and incidence of post-radiofrequency ablation syndrome: Prospective study. *Radiology* 2005; **237**: 1097–102.

36. Buscarini L, Buscarini E, Di Stasi M, *et al.* Percutaneous radiofrequency ablation of small hepatocellular carcinoma: Long-term results. *Eur Radiol* 2001; **11**: 914–21.

37. Lencioni R, Cioni D, Crocetti L, *et al.* Early-stage hepatocellular carcinoma in patients with cirrhosis: Long-term results of percutaneous image-guided radiofrequency ablation. *Radiology* 2005; **234**: 961–7.

38. Tateishi R, Shiina S, Teratani T, *et al.* Percutaneous radiofrequency ablation for hepatocellular carcinoma. An analysis of 1000 cases. *Cancer* 2005; **103**: 1201–9.

39. Guglielmi A, Ruzzenente A, Battocchia A, *et al.* Radiofrequency ablation of hepatocellular carcinoma in cirrhotic patients. *Hepato-Gastroenterology* 2003; **50**: 480–4.

40. Montorsi M, Santambrogio R, Bianchi P, *et al.* Survival and recurrences after hepatic resection of radiofrequency for hepatocellular carcinoma in cirrhotic patients: A multivariate analysis. *J Gastrointest Surg* 2005; **9**: 62–7.

41. Raut CP, Izzo F, Marra P, *et al.* Significant long-term survival after radiofrequency ablation of unresectable hepatocellular carcinoma in patients with cirrhosis. *Ann Surg Oncol* 2005; **12**: 616–28.

42. Chen MS, Li JQ, Zheng Y, *et al.* A prospective randomized trial comparing percutaneous local ablative therapy and partial hepatectomy for small hepatocellular carcinoma. *Ann Surg* 2006; **243**: 321–8.

43. Horiike N, Luchi H, Ninimiya T, *et al.* Influencing factor for recurrence for hepatocellular carcinoma treated with radiofrequency ablation. *Oncol Report* 2002; **9**: 1059–62.

44. Hori T, Nagata K, Hasuike S, *et al.* Risk factors for the local recurrence of hepatocellular carcinoma after a single session of percutaneous radiofrequency ablation. *J Gastroenterol* 2003; **38**: 977–81.

45. Lencioni RA, Allgaier HP, Cioni D, *et al.* Small hepatocellular carcinoma in cirrhosis: Randomized comparison of radiofrequency thermal ablation versus percutaneous ethanol injection. *Radiology* 2003; **228**: 235–40.

46. Harrison LE, Koneru B, Baramipour P, *et al.* Locoregional recurrences are frequent after radiofrequency ablation for hepatocellular carcinoma. *J Am Coll Surg* 2003; **197**: 759–64.

47. Lam VWT, Ng KKC, Chok KSH, *et al.* Risk factors and prognostic factors of local recurrence after radiofrequency ablation of hepatocellular carcinoma. *J Am Coll Surg* 2008; **207**: 20–9.

48. Yamanaka Y, Shiraki K, Muyashita K, *et al.* Risk factors for the recurrence of hepatocellular carcinoma after radiofrequency ablation of hepatocellular carcinoma in patients with hepatitis C. *World J Gastroenterol* 2005; **11**: 2174–8.

49. Komorizono Y, Oketani M, Sako K, *et al.* Risk factors for local recurrence of small hepatocellular carcinoma after a single session, single application of percutaneous radiofrequency ablation. *Cancer* 2003; **97**: 1253–62.

50. Lu DSK, Raman SS, Limanond P, *et al.* Influence of large peritumoral vessels on outcome of radiofrequency ablation of liver tumors. *J Vasc Interv Radiol* 2003; **14**: 12567–74.

51. Lu DSK, Yu NC, Raman SS, *et al.* Radiofrequency ablation of hepatocellular carcinoma: Treatment success as defined by histologic examination of the explanted liver. *Radiology* 2005; **234**: 954–60.

52. Kim YS, Rhim H, Lim HK, *et al.* Completeness of treatment in hepatocellular carcinomas treated with image-guided tumor therapies: Evaluation of positive predictive value of contrast-enhanced CT with histopathologic correlation in the explanted liver specimen. *J Comp Assist Tomogr* 2006; **30**: 578–82.

7.2 Systemic therapies for advanced hepatocellular carcinoma

a. Review of current status of radiotherapy for the treatment of hepatocellular carcinoma

Orit Gutfeld and Charlie Pan

Introduction

Historically, radiotherapy (RT) had an extremely limited role in the treatment of liver malignancies due to the low tolerance of the whole liver to radiation. The risk of radiation-induced liver disease (RILD) limits the dose that can be safely delivered to the whole liver to only 30–35 Gy in 2-Gy fractions [1], a dose that is well below the doses needed to eradicate solid tumors. The development of three-dimensional conformal RT (3-D CRT) allows the delivery of higher radiation doses to the tumor while minimizing the dose to the surrounding uninvolved liver. Advances in tumor targeting via improved diagnostic imaging, techniques to control or account for motion of the liver due to respiration, and the use of image guidance enable us to further escalate the dose to the tumor without increasing the toxicity.

Studies using modern RT techniques and higher doses for treating hepatocellular carcinoma (HCC) have shown encouraging results. The concepts of liver RT, the techniques, and the available clinical data will be reviewed in this chapter.

Liver tolerance to radiation

RILD may develop between 2 weeks to 4 months after hepatic irradiation and is characterized by anicteric hepatomegaly, ascites, and impaired liver function tests, occurring in the absence of disease progression. Serum alkaline phosphatase is typically markedly elevated, with only moderate elevations of liver transaminases and little or no increase in bilirubin. The underlying pathology is venoocclusive disease of the small liver veins with eventual atrophy of hepatocytes and liver fibrosis. The clinical outcome of RILD ranges from mild, reversible symptoms to progressive liver failure and death [1].

Primary Carcinomas of the Liver, ed. Hero K. Hussain and Isaac R. Francis. Published by Cambridge University Press. © Cambridge University Press 2010.

RILD develops in 5–10% of patients receiving 30–32 Gy to the whole liver in conventional fractionation, and this risk rises steeply with higher doses. However, in the era of 3-D CRT we need to quantify the partial liver tolerance to radiation rather than the whole organ tolerance. Similar to surgical experience showing that a portion of the liver can be safely resected, partial liver volumes can be safely irradiated to very high doses if a sufficient volume of the normal liver is spared. Three-dimensional planning provides quantitative tools for analyzing the relationship among the doses delivered, the liver volume irradiated, and the risk for RILD. An important step was the development of a mathematical model for prediction of normal-tissue complication probability (NTCP) based on dose–volume data [2]. The NTCP model enables individualizing the prescribed dose so that the patient receives the maximal possible dose for a given risk level based on the liver volume to be irradiated.

A series of prospective controlled studies at the University of Michigan has demonstrated the feasibility and safety of using the NTCP model to deliver doses well above the whole-liver tolerance dose to focal liver lesions [3,4,5]. Analysis of data from more than 200 patients treated in these studies established the parameters for the NTCP model and its validity [6]. The analysis also demonstrated a strong association between the mean liver dose and risk of RILD, with 5 and 50% RILD risk for mean liver doses of 32 and 40 Gy, respectively, in 1.5-Gy fractions given twice daily. Patients with primary hepatobiliary malignancies were found to have a lower tolerance to liver radiation compared to patients with liver metastases, a difference that reflects their underlying liver disease. It should be noted that patients with advanced cirrhosis (Child–Turcotte–Pugh [CTP] Class B and C) were excluded from these studies; therefore, these model parameters should not be used to estimate the risk of RILD in this population. Moreover, in patients with substantially altered liver function, other patterns of radiation-induced liver injury may occur, including exacerbation of preexisting hepatitis with markedly elevated transaminases or deteriorating liver function.

Studies from Asia have reported different model parameters than those found in Michigan [7,8,9]. Different patient populations, variations in the type and severity of the underlying liver disease, different fraction sizes and concurrent treatments, as well as variations in the definition of RILD, may explain these differences.

Other uncommon potential hepatic toxicities include biliary sclerosis and subcapsular injury.

Computed tomography (CT) and magnetic resonance imaging (MRI) following partial liver irradiation often demonstrate well-demarcated hypodense lesions corresponding to the radiation ports [10,11,12,13,14]. Dynamic contrast-enhanced imaging shows different enhancement patterns of the "radiation reaction" zone. These radiographic changes are reversible in most cases and do not correlate with clinical hepatic toxicity. However, differentiating these postradiation changes from recurrent tumor may be challenging [15]. Other radiographic changes are atrophy of the irradiated liver portion, liver volume loss, and compensatory hypertrophy of the non-irradiated liver regions.

Partial liver irradiation may cause radiation-induced injury to adjacent organs. In the above-mentioned trials at the University of Michigan, the most common severe complications were upper gastrointestinal ulceration and bleeding (5%) [5]. Other dose-limiting organs include the kidneys. A major portion of the right kidney may be within the high-dose region, and special care should be taken to spare the left kidney.

Three-dimensional conformal radiotherapy – technique

With CRT, accurate definition of the gross tumor volume (GTV) is crucial to avoid geographic misses and unnecessary irradiation of normal liver tissue. Yet, defining the GTV in the liver may be challenging. Voroney et al. reported significant differences between MRI-defined GTVs and CT-defined GTVs that can be large enough to alter highly conformal RT plans [16]. In the absence of radiologic-pathologic correlation data, they recommend that both triphasic CT scan and MRI scan be evaluated for GTV definition, as they both provide complementary information. The GTV is expanded to create clinical target volume (CTV) that includes areas of microscopic spread. The planning target volume (PTV) includes the CTV plus margins to allow for patient setup uncertainties (usually 0.5 cm) and liver respiratory motion (ranges between 0.5 and 3 cm in the craniocaudal dimension and should be determined individually for each patient based on fluoroscopy or four-dimensional CT). The margins needed for target motion can be significantly reduced by using strategies to control or compensate for respiratory motion, such as active breathing control [17], gated RT [18], or tumor tracking [19]. Patient setup uncertainties can be reduced by using better immobilization devices and image guidance at the time of treatment.

Three-dimensional CRT treatment plans are individualized and use multiple beams from different angles, including non-axial beams, to ensure PTV coverage

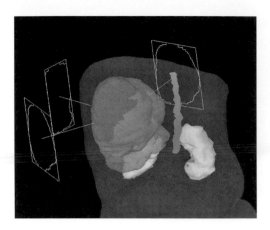

Figure 7.2a.1 Example of beam arrangement and field shapes used to treat a large HCC. The liver is shown in *gray*, PTV in *red*, kidneys in *yellow*, and spinal cord in *green*. (See color plate section.)

while maximally sparing the surrounding normal liver. An example of a typical beam arrangement with the resultant dose–volume histogram is provided in Figure 7.2a.1.

External beam radiotherapy – Clinical trials

The University of Michigan conducted Phase I and II trials in which 128 patients with unresectable hepatic malignancies were treated with CRT with concurrent continuous hepatic arterial floxuridine [5]. Of the 128 patients, 35 had HCC, 46 had intrahepatic cholangiocarcinoma (IHC), and 47 had liver metastases from colorectal cancer. RT was delivered in twice-daily 1.5-Gy fractions in two 2-week blocks separated by a 2-week break. The prescribed radiation dose was individualized so that each patient received the maximal possible dose associated with an estimated NTCP not exceeding 15%. Prescribed doses to the isocenter ranged from 40 Gy to 90 Gy (median 60.75 Gy). The median survival for HCC, cholangiocarcinoma, and metastatic colorectal cancer was 15.2, 13.3, and 17.2 months, respectively, which appears to be favorable when compared to historical controls. On multivariable analysis, the total radiation dose was found to be the only significant predictor of survival. Patients who received doses greater than or equal to 75 Gy had a significantly higher overall survival than those receiving lower doses had. RILD developed in five patients (4%). Pattern of failure analysis revealed a tendency of HCC tumors to progress locally, with 64% of recurrences occurring within the liver.

In a prospective Phase II French trial [20], 27 patients with small HCC (single nodule ≤5 cm or two nodules ≤3 cm each) of CTP Class A or B were treated with

Table 7.2a.1 Results of 3-D CRT in unresectable HCC

Study	No. of patients	CTP Class	PVT (%)	RT dose Total dose/fraction (Gy)	Response	Median survival after RT (months)	2-Year survival after RT
Park *et al.* [21]	59 (49 – salvage)	A– 56 B – 3	56%	30–55/2–3	66.1%	10	27.4%
Kim *et al.* [22]	70 (59 – salvage)	A– 56 B – 14	41%	44–54/2–3	54.3%	10.8	17.6%
Liu *et al.* [23]	44 (39 – salvage)	A– 32 B – 12	32%	39.6–60/1.8	61.4%	15.2 from diagnosis	40.3%

3-D CRT to 66 Gy in 2-Gy fractions. Fifteen of the patients had previously failed other treatments. Tumor response was observed in 92% of evaluable patients with complete response in 80%. Six patients (22%) developed in-field local recurrences with a median time to recurrence of 34 months. The majority of recurrences were in the liver outside the high-dose field, occurring at a median time of 7 months. In the CTP Class B patients, three patients (27%) developed acute grade 4 toxicity whereas no grade 4 or 5 acute or late toxicity was observed in the CTP Class A patients.

In addition to the above-mentioned prospective studies, retrospective series from Asia also support the safety and efficacy of 3-D CRT for HCC [21,22,23]. Most of the patients included in these studies had advanced-stage HCC (large tumors, portal vein thrombosis [PVT]), and many of them were unsuitable for other treatments or had failed other treatment modalities. The majority of patients had CTP Class A cirrhosis, but there was also representation of CTP Class B. Radiation dose ranged between 30 and 60 Gy in 1.8- to 3.0-Gy daily fractions. The objective tumor response ranged between 54 and 66%, with a median survival of 10 months. A dose–response relationship was found in some of these studies. The most prevalent pattern of failure was in the liver outside the radiation field. Toxicity was acceptable, with no cases of grade 4/5 toxicity. Transient, mildly abnormal liver function tests were seen in 43–70% of the patients 1 to 2 months after completion of treatment. Classic RILD was rare, but transient anicteric ascites without elevation of alkaline phosphatase was reported in 16 and 20% of the patients in two studies [21,22]. Some of these studies are summarized in Table 7.2a.1.

Overall, this experience suggests that high-dose RT to focal liver lesions may prolong survival of patients with large unresectable liver malignancies, who have limited treatment options.

External beam radiotherapy with transarterial chemoembolization

Transarterial chemoembolization (TACE) is a widely used non-surgical treatment modality that has proven to improve survival when compared to best supportive care in selected patients with unresectable HCC [24,25]. There is a large clinical experience, mainly from Asia, with combinations of TACE and RT that seems to offer better results compared to TACE alone [26,27,28,29,30]. Different strategies have been used, the most common being TACE followed by RT. In this approach, RT is delivered as a planned "consolidation" treatment that targets residual viable tumor after TACE. The iodized oil injection by TACE improves tumor delineation for RT by sharpening the GTV margin and highlighting previously unidentified lesions on post-TACE CT scan. Reduction of tumor volume after TACE may also allow less normal liver volume to be irradiated, thus permitting the use of higher doses with lower toxicity. However, as TACE decreases perfusion to the tumor, it may also result in areas of radioresistance due to hypoxia.

Another strategy is the use of RT either prior to TACE or after it to treat patients with unresectable HCC with PVT. TACE is less effective in the presence of PVT, and RT has been used in these studies to treat the PVT only [31,32,33].

Studies using TACE and RT are summarized in Table 7.2a.2. As shown, the reported objective responses range between 47 and 90%, with median survival of 10 to 25 months. The retrospective nature of these studies and the considerable variability in patient selection and treatment details make the interpretation of these results difficult. Nonetheless, this experience suggests a benefit of TACE and RT in advanced HCC compared to TACE alone.

Intensity-modulated radiotherapy

Intensity-modulated RT (IMRT) is another technological advancement that facilitates the delivery of highly conformal RT. With IMRT, radiation is delivered with multiple small fields within each beam (called "segments" or "beamlets"), each of which can be individually assigned radiation intensity. Thus, instead of delivering an almost homogenous dose profile over one large radiation field, the resulting

Table 7.2a.2 Selected results of RT with TACE in unresectable HCC

Study	No. of patients	CTP Class A/B	PVT (%)	Treatment radiation dose (Total dose/fraction), Gy	Response rate (%)	Median survival (months)
Seong *et al.* [26]	158	117/41	50.6	TACE + 25.2–60/1.8 or RT after TACE failure	67	10
Li *et al.* [27]	45	NR^a	33.3	TACE × 2 + 50.4/1.8 + TACE × 2	90	23.5
Guo *et al.* [28]	76	63/13	18.4	TACE + 30–50/1.8–2	47.4	19
Wu *et al.* [29]	94	43/51	NR	TACE + 48–60/4–7.5	90.5	25
Zeng *et al.* [30]	54	44/10	0	TACE + 36–60/2	76	20

^{a} NR, not reported.

delivered dose represents a highly complex map of varying radiation intensities from multiple beamlets. IMRT plans improve our ability to shape the dose and conform it to the target, allowing better normal tissue sparing and dose escalation to the tumor. In contrast, IMRT plans are more prone to uncertainties introduced by organ motion, as the dose gradients around the PTV are much steeper than conventional 3-D CRT plans. Because liver motion due to respiration may be quite large (average craniocaudal motion of 15.5 mm, range 6.9–35.4 mm) [34], strategies to control organ motion as well as image guidance should be implemented in conjunction with IMRT.

Planning studies have demonstrated the potential for dose escalation with IMRT for selected patients with liver malignancies [35,36,37], but clinical experience is still limited [38]. An example of a typical beam arrangement with the resultant dose–volume histogram is provided in Figure 7.2a.2.

Stereotactic body radiotherapy

Stereotactic body RT (SBRT) is an emerging treatment technique that provides precise targeting and dose delivery, allowing for potent ablative doses to be delivered to the target with either a single fraction or a small number of fractions. High degrees of dose conformality, attained by using multiple radiation fields, strategies to control or account for breathing motion, secure immobilization, accurate

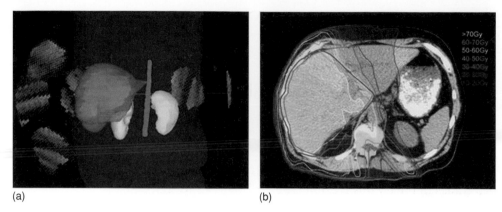

(a)   (b)

Figure 7.2a.2 (a and b) IMRT treatment for a patient with unresectable HCC. (a): Solid-surface reconstruction of the PTV (*red*), liver (*purple*), right and left kidneys (*yellow*), and the spinal cord (*green*) are shown, along with the projections of six IMRT fields, with the dose intensity in each beamlet represented by gray-scale. (b): Distribution of dose at the level of central axis. (See color plate section.)

repositioning, and the use of image guidance are all essential for the safe delivery of SBRT.

SBRT has been applied to patients with medically or surgically inoperable liver tumors, either primary or metastatic, and is usually limited to relatively small lesions (<6 cm). Based on surgical experience indicating that up to 80% of the liver volume can be safely removed, the mostly used dose constraint to the liver is that 700 ml or 35% of the normal liver volume (liver volume – GTV) should remain uninjured by SBRT.

There is limited literature on SBRT for primary liver malignancies. The first clinical experience with SBRT, reported by Blomgren *et al.*, included 9 HCC and 1 IHC patients with 20 lesions [39]. The minimum dose to the PTV varied from 15 to 45 Gy delivered in one to three fractions. Objective responses were seen in 70% and stable disease in 25%. Acute treatment-related toxicity was mild, but two patients developed intractable ascites within 6 weeks after therapy and subsequently expired. Subsequent studies focused mainly on patients with liver metastases and had only few patients with primary liver malignancies [40,41,42,43].

The largest experience with SBRT for primary liver cancer was published by Tse *et al.* [44]. In this Phase I study, an individualized iso-NTCP strategy was used to allocate patients to different dose levels according to the effective liver volume irradiated.

Data of 41 patients (31 HCC, 10 IHC) were reported. Twenty patients (49%) had vascular involvement. The median tumor volume was 173 ml with a range of

9 to 1913 ml. SBRT was given in six fractions with a median prescription dose of 36.0 Gy (24–54 Gy). Objective response was observed in 49% (complete response 5%, partial response 44%) and stable disease in 42%. The 1-year in-field local control was 65% (95% confidence interval, 44–79%). The most frequent site of first progression was in the liver outside the treated volume.

The median survival for all patients was 13.4 months with 1-year survival of 51%. For HCC and IHC, the median survival was 11.7 and 15 months with 1-year survival of 48 and 58%, respectively.

Overall, no dose-limiting toxicity or RILD was observed. Two patients with IHC had transient biliary obstruction during SBRT. Twenty-five percent of the patients developed grade 3 liver enzymes within the first 3 months after therapy, but no grade 4 or 5 liver enzymes changes were observed. The most clinically significant change after SBRT was a decline in CTP classification from A to B observed in seven patients (17%). These patients had higher median liver volume irradiated and higher mean liver doses.

The authors conclude that individualized six-fraction SBRT is safe and that the outcome is "better than expected," given the advanced disease of the patients.

Although liver SBRT is considered to be safe, the partial volume tolerance of the liver to SBRT is not well established, especially in patients with preexisting liver disease. Extrahepatic toxicities of liver SBRT have also been reported. These include gastritis, duodenal ulcers, colonic perforation, soft tissue and skin toxicity, and pleural effusions [45,46,47]. The dose constraints for adjacent normal tissues are not well established either.

In summary, SBRT is emerging as an additional treatment modality for selected patients with primary liver tumors. SBRT has potential radiobiological advantages of a short overall treatment time and high dose per fraction, together with other advantages such as decreased patient discomfort and increased department efficiency. SBRT also offers a non-invasive alternative for lesions in close proximity to vascular or biliary ductal structures that are not amenable to ablative procedures. In contrast, although initial data are promising, the experience with SBRT is still limited, and optimal fractionation schemes for HCC with background cirrhosis have to be investigated.

Proton beam and heavy ion therapy

The major advantage of high-energy protons and other heavy charged particles is their unique distribution of dose with depth. As the beam enters the body, there is a gentle incline in dose deposition along its path followed by a sharp peak (the

Table 7.2a.3 Selected results of proton beam and carbon ion RT for HCC

Study	No. of patients	CTP Class A/B/C (%)[a]	Tumor size median/range (cm)	Median total dose (range)/median fraction (range) (GyE)[b]	Local control rate	Survival
Chiba et al. [48]	162 (192 lesions)	50.6/38.3/6.2	3.8/1.5–14.5	72(50–88)/4.5 (2.9–6.0)	87% at 5 y	24% at 5 y
Kawashima et al. [49]	30	66.7/33.4/0	4.5/2.5–8.2	76/3.8	96% at 2 y	66% at 2 y
Hata et al. [50]	19	0/0/100	4/2.5–8.0	72(50–84)/3–5	95%	42% at 2 y
Bush et al. [51]	34	41/41 B+C	5.7/1.5–10	63/4.2	75% at 2 y	55% at 2 y
Kato et al. [52][c]	24	66.7/33.4/0	5/2.1–8.5	49.5–79.5/ 3.3–5.3	81% at 5 y	25% at 5 y

[a] The sum is less than 100% in certain cases because patients with no underlying liver disease were also included.

[b] GyE, cobalt Gray equivalent

[c] Carbon ion RT

Bragg peak), which is followed by a rapid falloff to zero. The high-dose region can be modulated to adapt to the tumor depth and thickness, and thus the dose is deposited within the target without exiting through normal tissues beyond it.

Based on the potential for better sparing of normal tissues, protons and carbon ion RT have been investigated as methods to deliver considerably higher RT doses to liver tumors [48,49,50,51,52]. A summary of selected studies is given in Table 7.2a.3. As shown, some of the best results of RT for HCC come from proton beam RT, with local control rates and 5-year survival as good as 87 and 25%, respectively. Unfortunately, at present, the high cost and limited availability of proton and carbon ion therapies hamper their common use.

Selective internal radiotherapy with radioactive isotopes

An alternative means of delivering focal radiation involves radioactive isotopes, either yttrium-90 (^{90}Y) embedded in glass or resin microspheres or iodine-131

(^{131}I)-labeled lipiodol, delivered selectively to the tumor via the hepatic artery. The dual blood supply of the liver is the basis for this "intra-arterial brachytherapy" or "radioembolization." Whereas liver malignancies derive most of their blood supply from the hepatic artery, normal liver tissue derives most of its blood supply from the portal system. Therefore, hepatic artery administration of radionuclides results in non-uniform dose distribution within the liver, with high radiation doses to the tumor and limited doses to the surrounding liver parenchyma. Compared with external beam RT, selective internal RT (SIRT) allows delivering considerably higher doses (100–150 Gy) to the tumor without significant liver toxicity. Clinical trials suggest that SIRT with ^{90}Y microspheres is safe and induces objective responses in patients with unresectable HCC [53,54,55,56]. In a series of 43 patients with HCC treated with ^{90}Y microspheres, 20 (47%) patients had an objective response, and median survival was 21 and 14 months for CTP Class A, and B and C, respectively. No life-threatening adverse events related to treatment were reported in this series [54]. The lack of large-scale prospective clinical trials using this technique makes it difficult to judge the efficacy and the role of this modality in the treatment of HCC. Current recommendations for its use have been published by the Radioembolization Brachytherapy Oncology Consortium [57].

Conclusions and future directions

With modern RT technology, high-dose CRT to liver lesions is feasible, with acceptable toxicity and promising results. Studies using high-dose RT for HCC have demonstrated high local control rates and improved survival compared to historical controls. A dose–response relationship was also demonstrated with improved outcomes in patients who received higher doses. Toxicity was strongly related to the baseline liver function and to the dose to the uninvolved liver.

RT has a potential role in a wide spectrum of HCC presentations. In early-stage disease, RT offers a non-invasive alternative for medically inoperable patients, especially for lesions that are not amenable to ablative procedures. In locally advanced unresectable HCC, RT in combination with regional or systemic therapies may serve as a definitive or palliative treatment.

However, most of the studies of RT for HCC are retrospective with variable patient selection criteria and a variety of treatment regimens and fractionation schemes. Prospective randomized trials are needed to better define the role of RT in HCC management and to better select the patients who are most likely to benefit from it. The optimal RT technique, fractionation, and combinations with other modalities should also be investigated in a prospective randomized manner.

The most prevalent pattern of failure following RT was in the liver outside the radiation field. Combining RT with liver-directed or systemic treatments may improve outcome and should be explored. The promising results with the targeted agent sorafenib in advanced HCC patients [58] make it an appealing candidate for such a combined approach [59]. Given the high vascularity of HCC, there is also a strong rationale for combining RT with agents (such as bevacizumab) that interfere with angiogencsis.

REFERENCES

1. Lawrence TS, Robertson JM, Anscher MS, Jirtle RL, Ensminger WD, and Fajardo LF. Hepatic toxicity resulting from cancer treatment. *Int J Radiat Oncol Biol Phys* 1995; **31**(5): 1237–48.

2. Lyman JT. Complication probability as assessed from dose-volume histograms. *Radiat Res Suppl* 1985; **8**: S13–19.

3. McGinn CJ, Ten Haken RK, Ensminger WD, Walker S, Wang S, and Lawrence TS. Treatment of intrahepatic cancers with radiation doses based on a normal tissue complication probability model. *J Clin Oncol* 1998; **16**(6): 2246–52.

4. Dawson LA, McGinn CJ, Normolle D, *et al.* Escalated focal liver radiation and concurrent hepatic artery fluorodeoxyuridine for unresectable intrahepatic malignancies. *J Clin Oncol* 2000; **18**(11): 2210–18.

5. Ben-Josef E, Normolle D, Ensminger WD, *et al.* Phase II trial of high-dose conformal radiation therapy with concurrent hepatic artery floxuridine for unresectable intrahepatic malignancies. *J Clin Oncol* 2005; **23**(34): 8739–47.

6. Dawson LA, Normolle D, Balter JM, McGinn CJ, Lawrence TS, and Ten Haken RK. Analysis of radiation-induced liver disease using the Lyman NTCP model. *Int J Radiat Oncol Biol Phys* 2002; **53**(4): 810–21.

7. Cheng JC, Wu JK, Lee PC, *et al.* Biologic susceptibility of hepatocellular carcinoma patients treated with radiotherapy to radiation-induced liver disease. *Int J Radiat Oncol Biol Phys* 2004; **60**(5): 1502–9.

8. Xu ZY, Liang SX, Zhu J, *et al.* Prediction of radiation-induced liver disease by Lyman normal-tissue complication probability model in three-dimensional conformal radiation therapy for primary liver carcinoma. *Int J Radiat Oncol Biol Phys* 2006; **65**(1): 189–95.

9. Liang SX, Zhu XD, Xu ZY, *et al.* Radiation-induced liver disease in three-dimensional conformal radiation therapy for primary liver carcinoma: The risk factors and hepatic radiation tolerance. *Int J Radiat Oncol Biol Phys* 2006; **65**(2): 426–34.

10. Yamasaki SA, Marn CS, Francis IR, Robertson JM, and Lawrence TS. High-dose localized radiation therapy for treatment of hepatic malignant tumors: CT findings and their relation to radiation hepatitis. *AJR Am J Roentgenol* 1995; **165**(1): 79–84.

11. Herfarth KK, Hof H, Bahner ML, *et al.* Assessment of focal liver reaction by multiphasic CT after stereotactic single-dose radiotherapy of liver tumors. *Int J Radiat Oncol Biol Phys* 2003; **57**(2): 444–51.

12. Chiou SY, Lee RC, Chi KH, Chia-Hsien Cheng J, Chiang JH, and Chang CY. The triple-phase CT image appearance of post-irradiated livers. *Acta Radiol* 2001; **42**(5): 526–31.

13. Ahmadi T, Itai Y, Onaya H, Yoshioka H, Okumura T, and Akine Y. CT evaluation of hepatic injury following proton beam irradiation: Appearance, enhancement, and 3D size reduction pattern. *J Comput Assist Tomogr* 1999; **23**(5): 655–63.

14. Onaya H, Itai Y, Yoshioka H, *et al.* Changes in the liver parenchyma after proton beam radiotherapy: Evaluation with MR imaging. *Magn Reson Imaging* 2000; **18**(6): 707–14.

15. Onaya H, Itai Y, Ahmadi T, *et al.* Recurrent hepatocellular carcinoma versus radiation-induced hepatic injury: Differential diagnosis with MR imaging. *Magn Reson Imaging* 2001; **19**(1): 41–6.

16. Voroney JP, Brock KK, Eccles C, Haider M, and Dawson LA. Prospective comparison of computed tomography and magnetic resonance imaging for liver cancer delineation using deformable image registration. *Int J Radiat Oncol Biol Phys* 2006; **66**(3): 780–91.

17. Eccles C, Brock KK, Bissonnette JP, Hawkins M, and Dawson LA. Reproducibility of liver position using active breathing coordinator for liver cancer radiotherapy. *Int J Radiat Oncol Biol Phys* 2006; **64**(3): 751–9.

18. Vedam SS, Keall PJ, Kini VR, and Mohan R. Determining parameters for respiration-gated radiotherapy. *Med Phys* 2001; **28**(10): 2139–46.

19. Shirato H, Shimizu S, Kitamura K, *et al.* Four-dimensional treatment planning and fluoroscopic real-time tumor tracking radiotherapy for moving tumor. *Int J Radiat Oncol Biol Phys* 2000; **48**(2): 435–42.

20. Mornex F, Girard N, Beziat C, *et al.* Feasibility and efficacy of high-dose three-dimensional-conformal radiotherapy in cirrhotic patients with small-size hepatocellular carcinoma non-eligible for curative therapies–mature results of the French phase II RTF-1 trial. *Int J Radiat Oncol Biol Phys* 2006; **66**(4): 1152–8.

21. Park W, Lim DH, Paik SW, *et al.* Local radiotherapy for patients with unresectable hepatocellular carcinoma. *Int J Radiat Oncol Biol Phys* 2005; **61**(4): 1143–50.

22. Kim TH, Kim DY, Park JW, *et al.* Three-dimensional conformal radiotherapy of unresectable hepatocellular carcinoma patients for whom transcatheter arterial chemoembolization was ineffective or unsuitable. *Am J Clin Oncol* 2006; **29**(6): 568–75.

23. Liu MT, Li SH, Chu TC, *et al.* Three-dimensional conformal radiation therapy for unresectable hepatocellular carcinoma patients who had failed with or were unsuited for transcatheter arterial chemoembolization. *Jpn J Clin Oncol* 2004; **34**(9): 532–9.

24. Llovet JM, Real MI, Montana X, *et al.* Arterial embolisation or chemoembolisation versus symptomatic treatment in patients with unresectable hepatocellular carcinoma: A randomised controlled trial. *Lancet* 2002; **359**(9319): 1734–9.

25. Lo CM, Ngan H, Tso WK, *et al.* Randomized controlled trial of transarterial lipiodol chemoembolization for unresectable hepatocellular carcinoma. *Hepatology* 2002; **35**(5): 1164–71.

26. Seong J, Park HC, Han KH, and Chon CY. Clinical results and prognostic factors in radiotherapy for unresectable hepatocellular carcinoma: A retrospective study of 158 patients. *Int J Radiat Oncol Biol Phys* 2003; **55**(2): 329–36.

27. Li B, Yu J, Wang L, *et al.* Study of local three-dimensional conformal radiotherapy combined with transcatheter arterial chemoembolization for patients with stage III hepatocellular carcinoma. *Am J Clin Oncol* 2003; **26**(4): e92–9.

28. Guo WJ and Yu EX. Evaluation of combined therapy with chemoembolization and irradiation for large hepatocellular carcinoma. *Br J Radiol* 2000; **73**(874): 1091–7.

29. Wu DH, Liu L, and Chen LH. Therapeutic effects and prognostic factors in three-dimensional conformal radiotherapy combined with transcatheter arterial chemoembolization for hepatocellular carcinoma. *World J Gastroenterol* 2004; **10**(15): 2184–9.

30. Zeng ZC, Tang ZY, Fan J, *et al.* A comparison of chemoembolization combination with and without radiotherapy for unresectable hepatocellular carcinoma. *Cancer J* 2004; **10**(5): 307–16.

31. Ishikura S, Ogino T, Furuse J, *et al.* Radiotherapy after transcatheter arterial chemoembolization for patients with hepatocellular carcinoma and portal vein tumor thrombus. *Am J Clin Oncol* 2002; **25**(2): 189–93.

32. Yamada K, Izaki K, Sugimoto K, *et al.* Prospective trial of combined transcatheter arterial chemoembolization and three-dimensional conformal radiotherapy for portal vein tumor thrombus in patients with unresectable hepatocellular carcinoma. *Int J Radiat Oncol Biol Phys* 2003; **57**(1): 113–19.

33. Lin CS, Jen YM, Chiu SY, *et al.* Treatment of portal vein tumor thrombosis of hepatoma patients with either stereotactic radiotherapy or three-dimensional conformal radiotherapy. *Jpn J Clin Oncol* 2006; **36**(4): 212–17.

34. Kirilova A, Lockwood G, Choi P, *et al.* Three-dimensional motion of liver tumors using cine-magnetic resonance imaging. *Int J Radiat Oncol Biol Phys* 2008; **71**(4): 1189–95.

35. Dvorak P, Georg D, Bogner J, Kroupa B, Dieckmann K, and Potter R. Impact of IMRT and leaf width on stereotactic body radiotherapy of liver and lung lesions. *Int J Radiat Oncol Biol Phys* 2005; **61**(5): 1572–81.

36. Cheng JC, Wu JK, Huang CM, *et al.* Dosimetric analysis and comparison of three-dimensional conformal radiotherapy and intensity-modulated radiation therapy for patients with hepatocellular carcinoma and radiation-induced liver disease. *Int J Radiat Oncol Biol Phys* 2003; **56**(1): 229–34.

37. Thomas E, Chapet O, Kessler ML, Lawrence TS, and Ten Haken RK. Benefit of using biologic parameters (EUD and NTCP) in IMRT optimization for treatment of intrahepatic tumors. *Int J Radiat Oncol Biol Phys* 2005; **62**(2): 571–8.

38. Fuss M, Salter BJ, Herman TS, and Thomas CR, Jr. External beam radiation therapy for hepatocellular carcinoma: Potential of intensity-modulated and image-guided radiation therapy. *Gastroenterology* 2004; **127**(5 Suppl 1): S206–17.

39. Blomgren H, Lax I, Naslund I, and Svanström R. Stereotactic high dose fraction radiation therapy of extracranial tumors using an accelerator. *Acta Oncol* 1995; **34**: 861–70.

40. Herfarth KK, Debus J, Lohr F, *et al.* Stereotactic single-dose radiation therapy of liver tumors: Results of a phase I/II trial. *J Clin Oncol* 2001; **19**: 164–70.

41. Herfarth KK, Debus J, and Wannenmacher M. Stereotactic radiation therapy of liver metastases: Update of the initial phase I/II trial. *Front Radiat Ther Oncol* 2004; **38**: 100–5.

42. Wulf J, Guckenberger M, and Haedinger U. Stereotactic radiotherapy of primary liver cancer and hepatic metastases. *Acta Oncol* 2006; **45**: 838–47.

43. Mendez Romero A, Wunderink W, Hussain SM, *et al.* Stereotactic body radiation therapy for primary and metastatic liver tumors: A single institution phase i-ii study. *Acta Oncol* 2006; **45**(7): 831–7.

44. Tse RV, Hawkins M, Lockwood G, *et al.* Phase I study of individualized stereotactic body radiotherapy for hepatocellular carcinoma and intrahepatic cholangiocarcinoma. *J Clin Oncol* 2008; **26**(4): 657–64.

45. Blomgren H, Ingmar L, Goranson H, *et al.* Radiosurgery for tumors in the body: Clinical experience using a new method. *J Radiosurg* 1998; **1**(1): 63 74.

46. Hoyer M, Roed H, Hansen AT, *et al.* Phase II study on stereotactic body radiotherapy for colorectal metastases. *Acta Oncol* 2006; **45**: 823–30.

47. Kavanagh BD, Schefter TE, Cardenes HR, *et al.* Interim analysis of a prospective phase I/II trial of SBRT for liver metastases. *Acta Oncol* 2006; **45**: 848–55.

48. Chiba T, Tokuuye K, Matsuzaki Y, *et al.* Proton beam therapy for hepatocellular carcinoma: A retrospective review of 162 patients. *Clin Cancer Res* 2005; **11**(10): 3799–805.

49. Kawashima M, Furuse J, Nishio T, *et al.* Phase II study of radiotherapy employing proton beam for hepatocellular carcinoma. *J Clin Oncol* 2005; **23**(9): 1839–46.

50. Hata M, Tokuuye K, Sugahara S, *et al.* Proton beam therapy for hepatocellular carcinoma patients with severe cirrhosis. *Strahlenther Onkol* 2006; **182**(12): 713–20.

51. Bush DA, Hillebrand DJ, Slater JM, and Slater JD. High-dose proton beam radiotherapy of hepatocellular carcinoma: Preliminary results of a phase II trial. *Gastroenterology* 2004; **127**(5 Suppl 1): S189–93.

52. Kato H, Tsujii H, Miyamoto T, *et al.* Results of the first prospective study of carbon ion radiotherapy for hepatocellular carcinoma with liver cirrhosis. *Int J Radiat Oncol Biol Phys* 2004; **59**(5): 1468–76.

53. Goin JE, Salem R, Carr BI, *et al.* Treatment of unresectable hepatocellular carcinoma with intrahepatic yttrium 90 microspheres: Factors associated with liver toxicities. *J Vasc Interv Radiol* 2005; **16**(2 Pt 1): 205–13.

54. Salem R, Lewandowski RJ, Atassi B, *et al.* Treatment of unresectable hepatocellular carcinoma with use of 90Y microspheres (TheraSphere): Safety, tumor response, and survival. *J Vasc Interv Radiol* 2005; **16**(12): 1627–39.

55. Lau WY, Leung WT, Ho S, *et al.* Treatment of inoperable hepatocellular carcinoma with intra-hepatic arterial yttrium-90 microspheres: A phase I and II study. *Br J Cancer* 1994; **70**(5): 994–9.

56. Kulik LM, Carr BI, Mulcahy MF, *et al.* Safety and efficacy of 90Y radiotherapy for hepatocellular carcinoma with and without portal vein thrombosis. *Hepatology* 2008; **47**(1): 71–81.

57. Kennedy A, Nag S, Salem R, *et al.* Recommendations for radioembolization of hepatic malignancies using yttrium-90 microsphere brachytherapy: A consensus panel report from the Radioembolization Brachytherapy Oncology Consortium. *Int J Radiat Oncol Biol Phys* 2007; **68**(1): 13–23.

58. Llovet J, Ricci S, Mazzaferro V, *et al.* Randomized phase III trial of sorafenib versus placebo in patients with advanced hepatocellular carcinoma (HCC). *J Clin Oncol* (Meeting Abstracts) 2007; **25**(18S): LBA1.

59. Tse RV, Guha C, and Dawson LA. Conformal radiotherapy for hepatocellular carcinoma. *Crit Rev Oncol Hematol* 2008; **67**(2): 113–23.

b. Review of current status of chemotherapy for the treatment of hepatocellular carcinoma

Edward Kim and Mark M. Zalupski

Hepatocellular carcinoma is the fifth most common cancer worldwide and the third most common cause of cancer death [1]. Viral hepatitis B and C are the major risk factors for hepatocellular carcinoma (HCC) leading to a roughly 20-fold increase in risk [2]. Heavy alcohol use and other toxin exposures, such as to aflatoxins, are also important risk factors [3]. Development of cirrhosis is the common link between these risk factors and the incidence of HCC. The high frequency of underlying cirrhosis in association with HCC creates difficulties in providing systemic treatment in the setting of impaired liver function. However, the historical ineffectiveness of treatment in advanced HCC is not limited simply to the challenge of giving systemic treatment in the setting of liver dysfunction. In this chapter, we discuss cytotoxic and biologic therapies that have been used in the past, and focus in greater detail on novel targeted agents that show promise in treatment of advanced HCC.

Cytotoxic agents

Chemotherapy has been extensively studied in an attempt to find an effective and tolerable treatment for advanced HCC. These efforts for the most part have been disappointing despite evaluating multiple chemotherapeutic agents and regimens. Overall, cytotoxic treatments have yielded objective response rates that are generally less than 20% with no significant impact on overall survival. Lack of efficacy is thought to be at least in part due to inherent and acquired drug resistance [4]. The chemotherapeutic drugs studied as single agents include the anthracyclines (doxorubicin [5,6], epirubicin [7,8], and mitoxantrone [9]), the antimetabolites (5-fluorouracil [5-FU] [10,11] and gemcitabine [12,13,14]), cisplatin [15], the topoisomerase inhibitors (irinotecan [16], topotecan [17], and etoposide [18]), and the taxanes [paclitaxel [19] and docetaxel [20]]. A recent Phase III trial

Primary Carcinomas of the Liver, ed. Hero K. Hussain and Isaac R. Francis. Published by Cambridge University Press. © Cambridge University Press 2010.

Table 7.2b.1 Phase III trials in HCC

	Doxorubicin vs. nolatrexed[5]		Doxorubicin vs. PIAF[3]4		Sorafenib vs. placebo[3]7	
	Doxorubicin $n = 222$	nolatrexed $n = 222$	Doxorubicin $n = 94$	PIAF $n = 94$	Sorafenib $n = 299$	placebo $n = 303$
Median overall survival (months)	8.1	5.6	6.8	8.7	10.7	7.9
Time to progression (months)	3.0	2.5	n/a	n/a	5.5	2.8
Response rate (%)	2.7	0.9	10.5	20.9	2.0	1.0

comparing an investigational thymidylate synthesis inhibitor (nolatrexed) to doxorubicin reported few objective responses and poor survival with both treatments [5] (Table 7.2b.1).

Attempts to increase response rates and improve survival have been made by combining two or more agents. However, with combination therapies, tolerance and safety become more of an issue as toxicity profiles are compounded. Doxorubicin, considered to be the single most active agent, has been combined with either gemcitabine or cisplatin and was tolerable, but unfortunately did not yield significant improvement in efficacy [21,22]. Other doublets studied in Phase II trials have included epirubicin and etoposide [23], cisplatin and 5-FU [24], cisplatin and gemcitabine [25], oxaliplatin and gemcitabine [26], and oxaliplatin and capecitabine [27]. Although some of these doublets have led to improved response rates, none has been shown to improve overall survival. Similarly, three drug combinations including an anthracycline, 5-FU or derivative, and cisplatin have generally demonstrated better response rates but failed to show a survival benefit and had varying additive toxicities [28,29,30,31]. Ultimately, systemic cytotoxic chemotherapy has not been demonstrated to provide substantial efficacy and therefore is not recommended as a standard treatment for advanced HCC.

Biotherapy

Interferons are a group of compounds with potent immunomodulatory effects as well as non-immunologic effects and have been tested as antineoplastic agents.

There has been conflicting evidence as to the efficacy of interferon as a single agent in treatment of HCC. A Chinese study comparing interferon to placebo [32] showed an improvement in response rate and median survival with minimal toxicity. In contrast, the Gastrointestinal Tumor Study Group (GITSG) found minimal response to interferon therapy and a high rate of significant toxicity [33]. Interferon has been combined with cytotoxic chemotherapy in a four-drug regimen including cisplatin, doxorubicin, and fluorouracil (PIAF). A Phase III trial of the PIAF regimen compared to doxorubicin as a single agent [34] yielded no statistical difference in overall survival and did have higher toxicity (Table 7.2b.1). Therefore, like cytotoxic chemotherapy, interferon is not a standard treatment for advanced HCC, either as a single agent or in combination with cytotoxic chemotherapy.

Targeted therapy

The review just mentioned illustrates the limitations of chemotherapy and biotherapy in the treatment of advanced HCC. Advances in the fundamental understanding of underlying tumor biology has ushered in a new era of molecular targeted therapies with a purported higher selectivity for cancer cells and the reciprocal ideal of less toxicity to normal tissues. Based on this increased understanding of the molecular targets relevant in the pathogenesis of hepatocellular cancer, several new agents are now therapeutic options.

The most promising novel agent is the multikinase inhibitor sorafenib, which was initially U.S. Food and Drug Administration (FDA) approved for treatment of renal cell carcinoma. Sorafenib is an oral agent with preclinical efficacy in various tumors via inhibition of several cellular kinases critical to tumor proliferation and angiogenesis. Sorafenib inhibits Raf kinase in the mitogen-activated protein kinase (MAPK) cascade, vascular endothelial growth factor receptors (VEGFRs) 2 and 3, and platelet-derived growth factor receptor (PDGFR)-beta [35,36]. Results from a Phase III trial comparing sorafenib and placebo were recently published [37]. Six hundred two patients with advanced hepatocellular cancer previously untreated systemically were randomized to receive either sorafenib or placebo. Median overall survival, the primary endpoint, was increased in the sorafenib group (10.7 vs. 7.9 months, $p < .0.001$) (Table 7.2b.1). This is the first robust and statistically significant improvement in overall survival in the treatment of advanced HCC, albeit the first placebo-controlled trial. Interestingly, there was minimal objective radiologic response in both groups, although the disease control rate, defined as the sum of complete and partial response plus stable disease, was higher in the sorafenib-treated group. Furthermore, sorafenib was relatively well tolerated with no significant difference in incidence of serious adverse events as compared to the placebo. The most frequent adverse events of any clinical consequence attributable to sorafenib included diarrhea, fatigue, and hand–foot syndrome, but these were limited to approximately or less than 10% of patients. This Phase III study restricted enrollment to patients with Child–Turcotte–Pugh (CTP) Class A, so the application of these findings to patients with more severe liver dysfunction is unknown. Based on these results demonstrating a statistically significant improvement in overall survival, sorafenib was granted approval in November 2007 for use in advanced HCC and is currently recognized as the standard first-line therapy in the treatment of this disease.

In addition to sorafenib, other targeted therapies are being tested in HCC. Sunitinib is a multikinase inhibitor, which (like sorafenib) was previously approved in renal cell carcinoma. It is a small molecule that inhibits VEGFRs 1 and 2 and PDGFR-alpha and -beta, as well as cKIT, Flt3, and RET kinases. A Phase II study demonstrated an encouraging median progression-free survival of 4.1 months but was associated with moderate toxicities including cytopenias, transaminitis, fatigue, and skin rash [38]. Erlotinib, a small molecule that binds to the kinase domain of endothelial growth factor receptor (EGFR) and prevents autophosphorylation, has yielded some disease control in two separate Phase II trials [39,40]. Cetuximab, a chimeric monoclonal antibody directed against EGFR, achieved similar results to erlotinib and was well tolerated, with skin rash the most frequent adverse event [41]. Cetuximab was combined with gemcitabine and oxaliplatin in a Phase II trial and yielded an encouraging median overall survival of 9.5 months [42].

Bevacizumab is a monoclonal antibody that targets circulating VEGF and is believed to affect angiogenesis. Phase 1 data using bevacizumab as a single agent suggested only mild activity in hepatocellular cancer [43]. Bevacizumab may provide synergistic activity with other therapies based on the hypothesis that it may normalize tumor vasculature [44]; thus it was tested in combination with gemcitabine and oxaliplatin. This three-drug regimen demonstrated modest effects on median overall survival (9.6 months) and progression-free survival (5.3 months) [45]. Bevacizumab was also combined with erlotinib with preliminary findings showing an encouraging response rate [46].

Further considerations and conclusions

The past 30 years of study of the treatment of advanced HCC has been marked by ineffective and toxic systemic bio- and chemotherapies. More recently, an improvement in overall survival achieved with sorafenib in a Phase III trial has defined a new era of systemic therapy for advanced HCC. Sorafenib is currently recommended as a standard-of-care, first-line therapy in this disease and will serve as a control arm in future clinical trials. Optimizing those clinical studies will require standardization in defining and targeting clinically relevant endpoints. This may be particularly relevant in the setting of the targeted therapies such as with sorafenib, where low objective radiologic response rates are observed despite improvements in survival. Furthermore, it will be important to select and stratify study patient populations with a standardized staging system to facilitate comparability between studies and to aid in determining applicability to clinical practice. The well-known CTP classification of liver dysfunction in cirrhosis can be used in the setting of HCC. However, the CTP classification was designed for cirrhosis only and does not incorporate tumor-specific characteristics limiting its utility in HCC. Several staging systems have been proposed that take the CTP classification or equivalent markers of liver function and variably add tumor-specific factors such as alpha-fetoprotein, tumor size, portal vein thrombosis, nodule number, and performance status. The Barcelona Clinic Liver Cancer (BCLC) classification includes the CTP criteria, performance status, tumor size, nodule number, and portal vein thrombosis. It has been prospectively validated [47,48] and is endorsed by both the American Association for the Study of Liver Diseases (AASLD) and the European Association for the Study of the Liver (EASL) [49,50]. The Cancer of Liver Italian Program (CLIP) scoring system was validated in Canada, Italy, and Japan [51,52,53] and was endorsed by a consensus conference of the American Hepato-Pancreato-Biliary Association and the American Joint Committee on Cancer (AHPBA/AJCC) [54]. These are two of the staging systems that have been applied sporadically in clinical trials, limiting their full utility in providing standardized and applicable information. The AASLD, therefore, recently recommended use of the BCLC staging system for both selection and stratification of patients for clinical trials [55]. It is hoped that this will further assist in the identification of new and effective therapies to add to the currently limited portfolio of effective systemic therapies for HCC.

REFERENCES

1. Parkin DM. Global cancer statistics in the year 2000. *Lancet Oncol* 2001; **2**: 533–43.
2. Donato F, Boffetta P, and Puoti M. A meta-analysis of epidemiological studies on the combined effect of hepatitis B and C virus infections in causing hepatocellular carcinoma. *Int J Cancer* 1998; **75**: 347–54.

3. El-Serag HB and Rudolph KL. Hepatocellular carcinoma: Epidemiology and molecular carcinogenesis. *Gastroenterology* 2007; **132**: 2557–76.

4. Huang CC, Wu MC, Xu GW, *et al.* Overexpression of the MDR1 gene and P-glycoprotein in human hepatocellular carcinoma. *J Natl Cancer Inst* 1992; **84**: 262–4.

5. Gish RG, Porta C, Lazar L, *et al.* Phase III randomized controlled trial comparing the survival of patients with unresectable hepatocellular carcinoma treated with nolatrexed or doxorubicin. *J Clin Oncol* 2007; **25**: 3069–75.

6. Lai CL, Wu PC, Chan GC, Lok AS, and Lin HJ. Doxorubicin versus no antitumor therapy in inoperable hepatocellular carcinoma. A prospective randomized trial. *Cancer* 1988; **62**: 479–83.

7. Colleoni M, Nole F, Di Bartolomeo M, de Braud F, and Bajetta E. Mitoxantrone in patients affected by hepatocellular carcinoma with unfavorable prognostic factors. *Oncology* 1992; **49**: 139–42.

8. Dobbs NA, Twelves CJ, Rizzi P, *et al.* Epirubicin in hepatocellular carcinoma: Pharmacokinetics and clinical activity. *Cancer Chemother Pharmacol* 1994; **34**: 405–10.

9. Pohl J, Zuna I, Stremmel W, and Rudi J. Systemic chemotherapy with epirubicin for treatment of advanced or multifocal hepatocellular carcinoma. *Chemotherapy* 2001; **47**: 359–65.

10. Porta C, Moroni M, Nastasi G, and Arcangeli G. 5-Fluorouracil and d,l-leucovorin calcium are active to treat unresectable hepatocellular carcinoma patients: Preliminary results of a phase II study. *Oncology* 1995; **52**: 487–91.

11. Tetef M, Doroshow J, Akman S, *et al.* 5-Fluorouracil and high-dose calcium leucovorin for hepatocellular carcinoma: A phase II trial. *Cancer Invest* 1995; **13**: 460–3.

12. Fuchs CS, Clark JW, Ryan DP, *et al.* A phase II trial of gemcitabine in patients with advanced hepatocellular carcinoma. *Cancer* 2002; **94**: 3186–91.

13. Guan Z, Wang Y, Maoleekoonpairoj S, *et al.* Prospective randomised phase II study of gemcitabine at standard or fixed dose rate schedule in unresectable hepatocellular carcinoma. *Br J Cancer* 2003; **89**: 1865–9.

14. Yang TS, Lin YC, Chen JS, Wang HM, and Wang CH. Phase II study of gemcitabine in patients with advanced hepatocellular carcinoma. *Cancer* 2000; **89**: 750–6.

15. Okada S, Okazaki N, Nose H, Shimada Y, Yoshimori M, and Aoki K. A phase 2 study of cisplatin in patients with hepatocellular carcinoma. *Oncology* 1993; **50**: 22–6.

16. Boige V, Taieb J, Hebbar M, *et al.* Irinotecan as first-line chemotherapy in patients with advanced hepatocellular carcinoma: A multicenter phase II study with dose adjustment according to baseline serum bilirubin level. *Eur J Cancer* 2006; **42**: 456–9.

17. Wall JG, Benedetti JK, O'Rourke MA, Natale RB, and Macdonald JS. Phase II trial to topotecan in hepatocellular carcinoma: A Southwest Oncology Group study. *Invest New Drugs* 1997; **15**: 257–60.

18. Wierzbicki R, Ezzat A, Abdel-Warith A, *et al.* Phase II trial of chronic daily VP-16 administration in unresectable hepatocellular carcinoma (HCC). *Ann Oncol* 1994; **5**: 466–7.

19. Chao Y, Chan WK, Birkhofer MJ, *et al.* Phase II and pharmacokinetic study of paclitaxel therapy for unresectable hepatocellular carcinoma patients. *Br J Cancer* 1998; **78**: 34–9.

20. Hebbar M, Ernst O, Cattan S, *et al.* Phase II trial of docetaxel therapy in patients with advanced hepatocellular carcinoma. *Oncology* 2006; **70**: 154–8.

21. Lee J, Park JO, Kim WS, *et al.* Phase II study of doxorubicin and cisplatin in patients with metastatic hepatocellular carcinoma. *Cancer Chemother Pharmacol* 2004; **54**: 385–90.

22. Yang TS, Wang CH, Hsieh RK, Chen JS, and Fung MC. Gemcitabine and doxorubicin for the treatment of patients with advanced hepatocellular carcinoma: A phase I-II trial. *Ann Oncol* 2002; **13**:1771–8.

23. Bobbio-Pallavicini E, Porta C, Moroni M, *et al.* Epirubicin and etoposide combination chemotherapy to treat hepatocellular carcinoma patients: A phase II study. *Eur J Cancer* 1997; **33**: 1784–8.

24. Tanioka H, Tsuji A, Morita S, *et al.* Combination chemotherapy with continuous 5-fluorouracil and low-dose cisplatin infusion for advanced hepatocellular carcinoma. *Anticancer Res* 2003; **23**: 1891–7.

25. Parikh PM, Fuloria J, Babu G, *et al.* A phase II study of gemcitabine and cisplatin in patients with advanced hepatocellular carcinoma. *Trop Gastroenterol* 2005; **26**: 115–18.

26. Louafi S, Boige V, Ducreux M, *et al.* Gemcitabine plus oxaliplatin (GEMOX) in patients with advanced hepatocellular carcinoma (HCC): Results of a phase II study. *Cancer* 2007; **109**: 1384–90.

27. Boige V, Raoul JL, Pignon JP, *et al.* Multicentre phase II trial of capecitabine plus oxaliplatin (XELOX) in patients with advanced hepatocellular carcinoma: FFCD 03–03 trial. *Br J Cancer* 2007; **97**: 862–7.

28. Boucher E, Corbinais S, Brissot P, Boudjema K, and Raoul JL. Treatment of hepatocellular carcinoma (HCC) with systemic chemotherapy combining epirubicin, cisplatinum and infusional 5-fluorouracil (ECF regimen). *Cancer Chemother Pharmacol* 2002; **50**: 305–8.

29. Ikeda M, Okusaka T, Ueno H, Takezako Y, and Morizane C. A phase II trial of continuous infusion of 5-fluorouracil, mitoxantrone, and cisplatin for metastatic hepatocellular carcinoma. *Cancer* 2005; **103**: 756–62.

30. Kim SJ, Seo HY, Choi JG, *et al.* Phase II study with a combination of epirubicin, cisplatin, UFT, and leucovorin in advanced hepatocellular carcinoma. *Cancer Chemother Pharmacol* 2006; **57**: 436–42.

31. Park SH, Lee Y, Han SH, *et al.* Systemic chemotherapy with doxorubicin, cisplatin and capecitabine for metastatic hepatocellular carcinoma. *BMC Cancer* 2006; **6**: 3.

32. Lai CL, Lau JY, Wu PC, *et al.* Recombinant interferon-alpha in inoperable hepatocellular carcinoma: A randomized controlled trial. *Hepatology* 1993; **17**: 389–94.

33. A prospective trial of recombinant human interferon alpha 2B in previously untreated patients with hepatocellular carcinoma. The Gastrointestinal Tumor Study Group. *Cancer* 1990; **66**: 135–9.

34. Yeo W, Mok TS, Zee B, *et al.* A randomized phase III study of doxorubicin versus cisplatin/interferon alpha-2b/doxorubicin/fluorouracil (PIAF) combination chemotherapy for unresectable hepatocellular carcinoma. *J Natl Cancer Inst* 2005; **97**: 1532–8.

35. Wilhelm SM, Carter C, Tang L, *et al.* BAY 43–9006 exhibits broad spectrum oral antitumor activity and targets the RAF/MEK/ERK pathway and receptor tyrosine kinases involved in tumor progression and angiogenesis. *Cancer Res* 2004; **64**: 7099–109.

36. Liu L, Cao Y, Chen C, *et al.* Sorafenib blocks the RAF/MEK/ERK pathway, inhibits tumor angiogenesis, and induces tumor cell apoptosis in hepatocellular carcinoma model PLC/PRF/5. *Cancer Res* 2006; **66**: 11851–8.

37. Llovet JM, Ricci S, Mazzaferro V, *et al.* Sorafenib in advanced hepatocellular carcinoma. *N Engl J Med* 2008; **359**: 378–90.

38. Zhu AX, Sahani DV, di Tomaso E, *et al.* A phase II study of sunitinib in patients with advanced hepatocellular carcinoma. *J Clin Oncol* 2007; **25**: Abstract 4637.

39. Thomas MB, Chadha R, Glover K, *et al.* Phase 2 study of erlotinib in patients with unresectable hepatocellular carcinoma. *Cancer* 2007; **110**: 1059–67.

40. Philip PA, Mahoney MR, Allmer C, *et al.* Phase II study of Erlotinib (OSI-774) in patients with advanced hepatocellular cancer. *J Clin Oncol* 2005; **23**: 6657–63.

41. Zhu AX, Stuart K, Blaszkowsky LS, *et al.* Phase 2 study of cetuximab in patients with advanced hepatocellular carcinoma. *Cancer* 2007; **110**: 581–9.

42. Asnacios A, Fartoux L, Romano O, *et al.* Gemcitabine plus oxaliplatin (GEMOX) combined with cetuximab in patients with progressive advanced stage hepatocellular carcinoma: Results of a multicenter phase 2 study. *Cancer* 2008; **112**(12): 2733–9.

43. Schwartz JD, Schwartz M, Lehrer D, *et al.* Bevacizumab in unresectable hepatocellular carcinoma (HCC) for patients without metastasis and without invasion of the portal vein. *J Clin Oncol* 2006; **24**: Abstract 4144.

44. Jain RK. Normalizing tumor vasculature with anti-angiogenic therapy: A new paradigm for combination therapy. *Nat Med* 2001; **7**: 987–9.

45. Zhu AX, Blaszkowsky LS, Ryan DP, *et al.* Phase II study of gemcitabine and oxaliplatin in combination with bevacizumab in patients with advanced hepatocellular carcinoma. *J Clin Oncol* 2006; **24**: 1898–903.

46. Thomas MB, Chadha R, Iwasaki M, Glover K, and Abbruzzese JL. The combination of bevacizumab (B) and erlotinib (E) shows significant biological activity in patients with advanced hepatocellular carcinoma (HCC). *J Clin Oncol* 2007; **25**: Abstract 4567.

47. Cillo U, Vitale A, Grigoletto F, *et al.* Prospective validation of the Barcelona Clinic Liver Cancer staging system. *J Hepatol* 2006; **44**: 723–31.

48. Marrero JA, Fontana RJ, Barrat A, *et al.* Prognosis of hepatocellular carcinoma: Comparison of 7 staging systems in an American cohort. *Hepatology* 2005; **41**: 707–16.

49. Bruix J and Sherman M. Management of hepatocellular carcinoma. *Hepatology* 2005; **42**: 1208–36.

50. Bruix J, Sherman M, Llovet JM, *et al.* Clinical management of hepatocellular carcinoma. Conclusions of the Barcelona-2000 EASL conference. European Association for the Study of the Liver. *J Hepatol* 2001; **35**: 421–30.

51. Levy I and Sherman M. Staging of hepatocellular carcinoma: Assessment of the CLIP, Okuda, and Child-Pugh staging systems in a cohort of 257 patients in Toronto. *Gut* 2002; **50**: 881–5.

52. Farinati F, Rinaldi M, Gianni S, and Naccarato R. How should patients with hepatocellular carcinoma be staged? Validation of a new prognostic system. *Cancer* 2000; **89**: 2266–73.

53. Ueno S, Tanabe G, Sako K, *et al.* Discrimination value of the new western prognostic system (CLIP score) for hepatocellular carcinoma in 662 Japanese patients. Cancer of the Liver Italian Program. *Hepatology* 2001; **34**: 529–34.

54. Helton W and Strasberg S. AHPBA/AJCC consensus conference on staging of hepatocellular carcinoma: Rationale and overview of the conference. *HPB* (Oxford) 2003; **5**: 238–42.

55. Llovet JM, Di Bisceglie AM, Bruix J, *et al.* Design and endpoints of clinical trials in hepatocellular carcinoma. *J Natl Cancer Inst* 2008; **100**: 698–711.

8

Radiological identification of residual and recurrent hepatocellular carcinoma

Peter S. Liu, Ajaykumar C. Morani, and Hero K. Hussain

Minimally invasive techniques, including thermal ablation and transarterial chemo-embolization (TACE), for the management of hepatocellular carcinoma (HCC) have evolved substantially over the past decade. Although surgical techniques remain the best curative option for HCC, many patients are poor surgical candidates due to severe hepatic dysfunction, comorbid conditions, or extent of tumor burden [1]. Minimally invasive therapies are being used more frequently as an alternative primary treatment option, with either a palliative or curative intent [1,2]. Critical to the management of such patients is the posttreatment imaging that is tasked with detecting residual disease and facilitating early detection of recurrent disease. This chapter discusses the computed tomography (CT) and magnetic resonance imaging (MRI) appearances of patients who have undergone minimally invasive therapy for HCC, including ablation and TACE, with an emphasis on the normal posttreatment appearance and features of residual and recurrent disease. Although both CT and MRI are used for the assessment of residual and recurrent disease, the practice in our hospital is to use MRI for postprocedural follow-up.

Background

The prompt identification of residual or recurrent disease may facilitate additional successful intervention at an early stage [3]. Additionally, posttreatment imaging may also reveal postprocedural complications such as hepatic abscess, localized biliary ductal dilation, or biloma. Traditionally, the efficacy of treatment for cancer has been measured by criteria proposed by the World Health Organization (WHO), which use the morphological changes in a lesion's size as a marker of treatment success or failure [4]. Because of the extensive local tumor necrosis and associated scarring that occurs during both ablative and transarterial therapies, the

Primary Carcinomas of the Liver, ed. Hero K. Hussain and Isaac R. Francis. Published by Cambridge University Press. © Cambridge University Press 2010.

treatment bed often is slow to decrease in size, despite histological proof of tumor necrosis [5,6]. Furthermore, many thermal ablation techniques are performed with a safety margin of 0.5 to 1.0 cm incorporated into the expected treatment volume [7]. Therefore, the use of treatment zone size as a proxy for therapeutic efficacy may be inaccurate after local ablative or transarterial techniques. Early contrast enhancement (in the arterial phase) within a treatment zone suggests the persistence of viable tumor, and although nonspecific, it has been used as an additional marker for treatment efficacy besides morphology [8]. As a result, the use of contrast-enhanced tomographic techniques has been advocated after percutaneous treatment, because both morphology and enhancement can be evaluated in a single method [8,9]. Newer techniques looking at other non-morphologic features of a treatment zone, such as diffusion-weighted MRI, have demonstrated mixed results to date [10,11].

Protocol

With the advent of multidetector CT and modern MRI sequences, high-resolution imaging can be obtained in relatively short periods of time. The specific imaging protocol used in patients after minimally invasive therapy varies by institution, including the timing of follow-up imaging. From a general standpoint, several key protocol concepts are ubiquitous. For CT, several sources advocate the use of a multiphase protocol, which includes non-contrast images and several contrast-enhanced sequences, which were obtained during the arterial, venous, and equilibrium phases of hepatic enhancement (30, 70, and 180–300 seconds after injection, respectively) [5,8]. For MRI, the basic sequences required include a T2-weighted (T2W) sequence, precontrast T1-weighted (T1W) sequence, and a dynamic (multiphase) postcontrast T1W sequence [5,8]. Some authors have suggested using a high resolution, respiratory triggered T2W sequences to optimize lesion detection and lessen the impact of respiratory motion [5].

Additionally, the actual timing of follow-up imaging varies by institution. Most authors agree that a short-term imaging follow-up is required; it is often obtained at 1 to 2 months after the procedure [5,8]. An immediate postprocedural scan is variably employed – several authors have suggested a role for contrast-enhanced ultrasound as an option for immediate postprocedural scanning [7,8]. Subsequent examinations are usually performed every 3 to 6 months. At some institutions, the duration of time between scans will be increased if the patient shows no residual or recurrent disease on several serial examinations.

Imaging after ablative therapy

There are a variety of local ablative techniques that can be used for the treatment of HCC, including thermal ablative techniques (such as radiofrequency ablation [RFA], microwave ablation, or cryoablation) and direct injection of a cytotoxic compound (such as absolute ethanol) into the tumor. The net result of such therapy is localized coagulation necrosis, resulting in avascular tissue [3]. Additionally, the increasing use of ablation techniques for smaller lesions places an emphasis on excellent spatial resolution to accurately define the treatment zone. Studies have shown that contrast-enhanced CT and MRI can accurately delineate the treatment bed to within 2 mm [5,9]. Therefore, contrast-enhanced CT or MRI is appropriate for follow-up imaging of patients after local ablation procedures.

The normal posttreatment appearance of an ablation zone on CT can vary depending on the time since prior treatment. The non-contrast CT appearance of an ablation zone is generally hypodense versus adjacent hepatic parenchyma, but can have foci of heterogeneous internal hyperattenuation related to coagulation necrosis on the early posttreatment study at 1 to 2 months [5]. Because of the safety zone that is incorporated into the treatment volume, the actual size of the treatment zone may be larger than the preprocedure lesion itself. Some authors have suggested that, if the size of the initial postablation zone is not larger than the pretreatment lesion size, close attention must be paid for possible local residual or early recurrent disease [8]. On contrast-enhanced imaging, there should be no internal enhancement within the treatment zone, including on early posttreatment studies [3]. The presence of thin-rim enhancement around the treatment site on the initial posttreatment study (1–2 months) represents reactive hyperemia or inflammatory reaction to the coagulative necrosis induced by local ablation [5,8]. This inflammatory rim is uniform in size, approximately 1 mm or less in thickness, and remains either isoattenuating or hyperattenuating to background hepatic parenchyma on later phases of dynamic imaging [5,8]. This inflammatory rim often resolves on subsequent follow-up studies, generally by 6–12 months [5]. Small, non-tumorous, geometric, wedge-shaped foci of enhancement, which have been attributed to iatrogenic areas of arterial-venous shunting, have also been reported adjacent to the treatment bed or needle track [3,8]. These foci have been reported in up to 12% of patients in one series [5]. These shunts are usually easily seen on arterial phase imaging, with near-isointensity on later phases of dynamic imaging. Often, these foci will resolve over time as well, with one series reporting resolution of all vascular shunts by 6 months [5]. Therefore, not all enhancement around the ablation

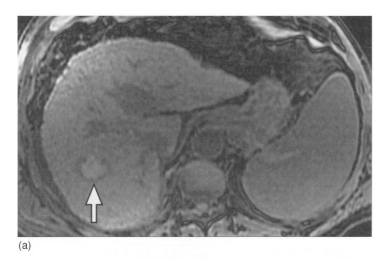

(a)

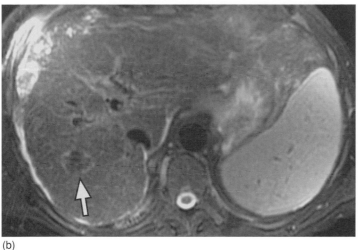

(b)

Figure 8.1 (a–d) Successfully ablated HCC in the posterior right lobe. The RFA cavity (*arrow*) is high in signal intensity on T1W imaging (a) and hypointense on T2W imaging (b) relative to liver parenchyma due to coagulative necrosis. There is no enhancement with the cavity in the arterial phase (c) or on subtraction imaging (d). A thin rim of enhancement (d, *arrowhead*) around the cavity in the arterial phase is postprocedural.

site on CT should be considered tumor, particularly on the early posttreatment studies [8].

The normal posttreatment appearance of an ablation zone on MRI is also highly variable depending on the time since prior treatment. Because of coagulation necrosis, unenhanced MRI can show regions of increased signal intensity on both T1- and T2W sequences (Figure 8.1a). In one series, 28% of treatment zones were low

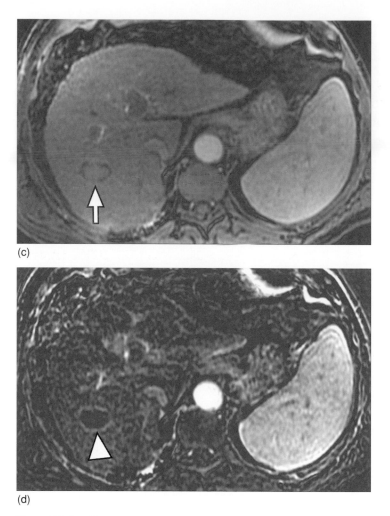

(c)

(d)

Figure 8.1 (cont.)

signal intensity on T1W imaging, whereas 72% demonstrated some heterogeneity, often with a peripheral ring of increased signal intensity [5]. T2W sequences demonstrated even more variety, with the majority of treatment zones showing homogeneous hypointensity (attributed to the dehydrating effect of thermal ablation) (Figure 8.1b), although isointense and even markedly hyperintense signal intensities were also reported [3,5]. The normal contrast-enhanced MRI appearance also mimics that of contrast-enhanced CT, in that no internal enhancement is typically seen on any of the studies (Figure 8.1c). Because of the intrinsic increased signal on T1W images related to coagulation necrosis, subtle areas of enhancement on postcontrast T1W images may be hard to detect without the use of subtraction data sets (Figure 8.1d). The inflammatory rim and arteriovenous shunts seen on contrast-enhanced CT have also been reported on MRI (Figure 8.1, c and d), with similar morphologic and enhancement characteristics [3,8].

Residual or recurrent disease in the setting of prior ablation generally has similar characteristics on both CT and MRI. Morphologically, residual or recurrent disease can have two different forms. In the first form, there may be one or several small nodules (5–15 mm) located eccentrically around a treatment zone, often with marginal contact with the treatment bed itself [5,8]. On CT, these nodules are best revealed on contrast-enhanced sequences where they enhance conspicuously on arterial phase imaging versus the hypovascular treatment zone, and can demonstrate subsequent intralesional hypoattenuation on later phases of dynamic imaging [3]. Because of the multiple sequences available on MRI, lesion detection is predicated on both the T2W and postcontrast T1W appearance. On T2W images, such tumor nodules are often hyperintense to the treatment zone and minimally hyperintense to the hepatic parenchyma; however, the degree of hyperintensity is intermediate, and not as hyperintense as simple fluid such as cerebrospinal fluid or bile [5]. On dynamic contrast-enhanced MRI, the nodules will demonstrate a similar enhancement pattern to contrast-enhanced CT (Figure 8.2). The second pattern of disease is an irregular thickened rim (4–5 mm) around the ablation site, which demonstrates similar enhancement and signal characteristics on CT and MRI as the isolated tumor nodules (Figure 8.3) [5,8]. It has been suggested that MRI may be superior to CT in the detection of residual and recurrent disease due to the sensitivity of T2W sequences that exploit the tissue contrast differences between viable tumor and the necrotic ablation bed [1,3,8]. In one study looking at the efficacy of each modality, the reported sensitivity and specificity for tumor detection of MRI at 2 months were reported as 89% and 100%, respectively, versus a reported sensitivity of 44% and specificity of 100% by CT at 2 months [5].

Beyond morphology and enhancement characteristics, the temporal stability of a lesion across serial examinations is another valuable tool to assess for residual or recurrent disease. The ablation site may remain stable in size across several examinations or show a gradual decrease in size, thought to represent contraction of a necrotic or fibrotic zone [8]. Over long periods of time, a measurable decrease may be detected; one series reported a 15% decrease in size at 6 months and a 35% decrease in size at 12 months [5]. An increase in size should be viewed with concern for residual or recurrent tumors [8].

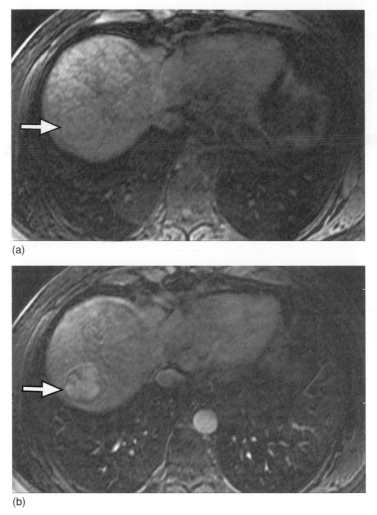

(a)

(b)

Figure 8.2 (a–e) A 4-cm HCC (*arrow*) in the dome of the liver, before and after RFA. The tumor is isointense to liver parenchyma on precontrast T1W three-dimensional gradient-echo imaging (a), hypervascular in the arterial phase of enhancement (b), and hypointense ("washes-out") at delayed postcontrast imaging (c). Following RFA, there is a large area of residual enhancement in the posterior aspect of the cavity (*arrowhead*) in the arterial phase (d) confirmed on subtraction imaging (e) indicating residual tumor.

Imaging after transarterial therapy

TACE as a primary therapy for inoperable HCC has been validated as a palliative measure to increase patient survival [12]. Because the therapeutic approach targets a selective or superselective vascular territory, the margins of the treatment bed are

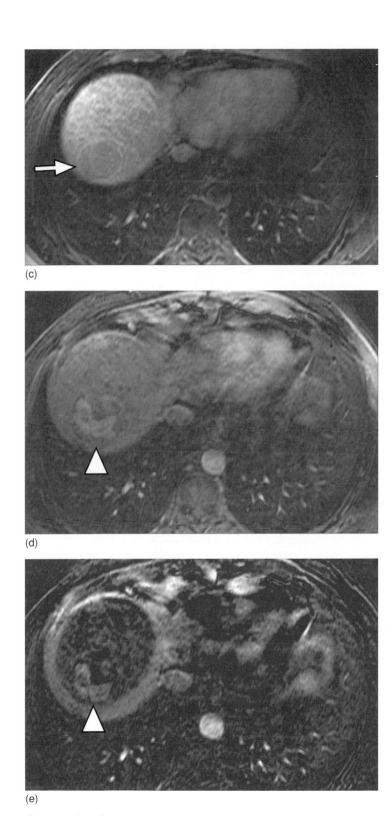

(c)

(d)

(e)

Figure 8.2 (*cont.*)

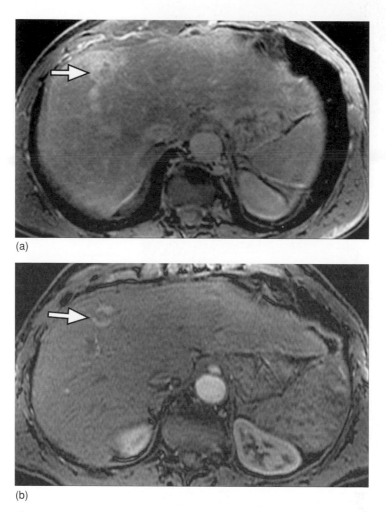

(a)

(b)

Figure 8.3 (a–g) A 2-cm HCC in the anterior right lobe, before and after two sessions of TACE. The tumor (*arrow*) is ill defined and hypervascular in the arterial phase of enhancement (a). Following the first TACE, the nodular rim enhancement (*arrow*) at the periphery of the cavity in the arterial phase (b) is confirmed on subtraction imaging (arterial – precontrast) (c), indicating residual tumor. The residual tumor (*arrow*) increased in size 3 months later as on arterial phase imaging (d). Following a second session of TACE, the cavity (*arrow*) is high in signal intensity on precontrast T1W imaging relative to liver parenchyma (e), but no enhancement is seen about the cavity (*arrow*) in the arterial phase (f). This is confirmed on subtraction imaging (g), indicating complete response to treatment.

less well delineated than in thermal ablation. Prior to the use of iodized oil as a vehicle for delivering chemotherapeutic agents, the postprocedural evaluation for residual or recurrent tumor was relatively straightforward, relying on the use of multiphase CT to demonstrate residual, viable areas of tumor as enhancing foci

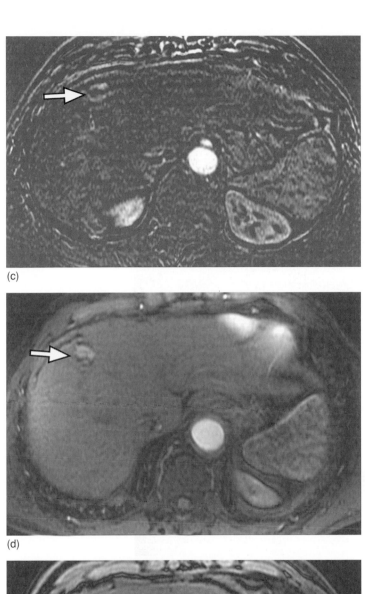

(c)

(d)

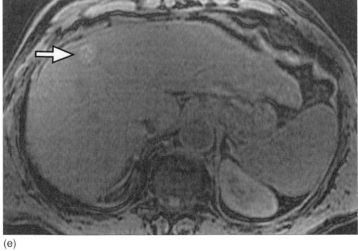

(e)

Figure 8.3 (*cont.*)

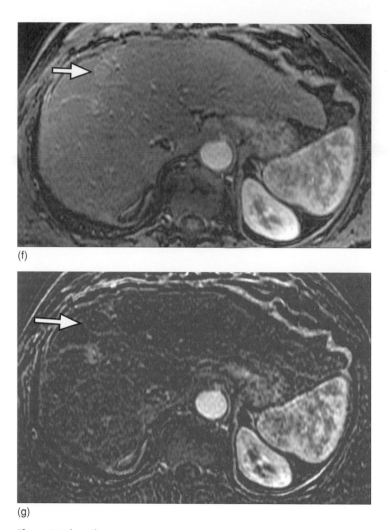

(f)

(g)

Figure 8.3 (*cont.*)

[13]. However, with the advent of modern techniques that frequently use iodized oil in the chemoembolization mixture, the postprocedural evaluation has become more difficult on CT due to the intrinsic high attenuation of retained iodized oil [6]. In patients who have received iodized oil, several follow-up imaging strategies have been discussed. On noncontrast CT, the retained iodized oil will remain hyperattenuating versus the background unenhanced liver. Focal defect or washout of iodized oil within a treated area suggests the presence of viable tumor [14]. Histopathologic studies have shown near-complete tumor necrosis (98% mean necrosis rate) in regions that have complete iodized oil uptake, as opposed to

partial necrosis in areas of incomplete iodized oil uptake (64% necrosis rate) [15]. However, areas of intratumoral necrosis also do not retain iodized oil, and thus may be a source of false-positive results on follow-up non-contrast CT [3]. The use of multiphase CT (including pre- and dynamic postcontrast imaging) has been described, with success in measuring quantitative changes of at least 20 Hounsfield units in the iodized oil–deficient areas on precontrast and postcontrast imaging [16]. The use of contrast enhancement would aid in the differentiation of viable tumor from intratumoral necrotic foci, which is problematic on non-contrast imaging alone. However, these data demonstrate some size bias that may limit practical application, as patients with HCCs less than 3 cm and those with small, iodized oil–deficient areas (<1 cm) were all excluded from the study population [16].

As a result of perceived difficulties in identifying residual or recurrent disease on CT, MRI has been proposed for postprocedural evaluation of patients with prior TACE. On T2W images and precontrast T1W images, there can be substantial heterogenous signal intensity, ascribed to intratumoral hemorrhage and coagulation necrosis [3,14]. There has been substantial debate on the effect of retained iodized oil on T1W and T2W images. It has been reported to decrease T1 and increase T2 relaxation times in lymph nodes when used in lymphangiography [17]. However, others have suggested that the concentration of iodized oil in the treatment bed is too low to modify the signal characteristics after some small time delay (varying between 1 and 11 weeks) from the chemoembolization procedure itself [18]. Foci of signal loss on out-of-phase imaging relative to in-phase have been reported at the site of lipiodol uptake owing to the lipid content [19]. The use of dynamic contrast enhancement on MRI has been shown to be effective in delineating residual or recurrent disease, with a reported sensitivity and specificity of 100% each; however, in this study, only 83% of all lesions were evaluated on dynamic contrast-enhanced MRI due to intrinsic high signals on precontrast images [18]. Presumably, the use of subtraction data sets would aid in increasing the percentage of lesions to which dynamic contrast-enhanced MRI could be applied.

In summary, both CT and MRI are effective in assessing residual and recurrent disease after therapy. We use MRI for posttherapy assessment at our institution. Residual tumor has signal and enhancement characteristics similar to those of the original tumor. Subtraction imaging is often necessary, especially after RFA, to distinguish coagulative necrosis from residual tumor. A persistent rim of inflammatory enhancement is often seen around the treatment cavity and should not be mistaken for residual tumor. New techniques such as diffusion-weighted imaging are currently being studied to assess tumor response to minimally invasive therapy.

REFERENCES

1. Sironi S, Livraghi T, Meloni F, De Cobelli F, Ferrero C, and Del Maschio A. Small hepatocellular carcinoma treated with percutaneous RF ablation: MR imaging follow-up. *AJR Am J Roentgenol* 1999 Nov; **173**(5): 1225–9.

2. Chung YH. A strategy for early detection of recurrent hepatocellular carcinoma following initial remission by transcatheter arterial chemoembolization. *Intervirology* 2005; **48**(1): 46–51.

3. Guan YS, Sun L, Zhou XP, Li X, and Zheng XH. Hepatocellular carcinoma treated with interventional procedures: CT and MRI follow-up. *World J Gastroenterol* 2004; **10**(24): 3543–8.

4. Miller AB, Hoogstraten B, Staquet M, and Winkler A. Reporting results of cancer treatment. *Cancer* 1981; **47**(1): 207–14.

5. Dromain C, de Baere T, Elias D, *et al.* Hepatic tumors treated with percutaneous radio-frequency ablation: CT and MR imaging follow-up. *Radiology* 2002; **223**(1): 255–62.

6. Takayasu K, Arii S, Matsuo N, *et al.* Comparison of CT findings with resected specimens after chemoembolization with iodized oil for hepatocellular carcinoma. *AJR Am J Roentgenol* 2000; **175**(3): 699–704.

7. Lencioni R, Della Pina C, and Bartolozzi C. Percutaneous image-guided radiofrequency ablation in the therapeutic management of hepatocellular carcinoma. *Abdom Imaging* 2005; **30**(4): 401–8.

8. Kim SK, Lim HK, Kim YH, *et al.* Hepatocellular carcinoma treated with radio-frequency ablation: Spectrum of imaging findings. *Radiographics* 2003; **23**(1): 107–21.

9. Solbiati L, Ierace T, Goldberg SN, *et al.* Percutaneous US-guided radio-frequency tissue ablation of liver metastases: Treatment and follow-up in 16 patients. *Radiology* 1997; **202**(1): 195–203.

10. Goshima S, Kanematsu M, Kondo H, *et al.* Evaluating local hepatocellular carcinoma recurrence post-transcatheter arterial chemoembolization: Is diffusion-weighted MRI reliable as an indicator? *J Magn Reson Imaging* 2008; **27**(4): 834–9.

11. Kamel IR, Bluemke DA, Ramsey D, *et al.* Role of diffusion-weighted imaging in estimating tumor necrosis after chemoembolization of hepatocellular carcinoma. *AJR Am J Roentgenol* 2003; **181**(3): 708–10.

12. Llovet JM and Bruix J. Systematic review of randomized trials for unresectable hepatocellular carcinoma: Chemoembolization improves survival. *Hepatology* 2003; **37**(2): 429–42.

13. Takayasu K, Moriyama N, Muramatsu Y, *et al.* Hepatic arterial embolization for hepatocellular carcinoma. Comparison of CT scans and resected specimens. *Radiology* 1984; **150**(3): 661–5.

14. Lim HS, Jeong YY, Kang HK, Kim JK, and Park JG. Imaging features of hepatocellular carcinoma after transcatheter arterial chemoembolization and radiofrequency ablation. *AJR Am J Roentgenol* 2006; **187**(4): W341–9.

15. Choi BI, Kim HC, Han JK, *et al.* Therapeutic effect of transcatheter oily chemoembolization therapy for encapsulated nodular hepatocellular carcinoma: CT and pathologic findings. *Radiology* 1992; **182**(3): 709–13.

16. Kim SH, Lee WJ, Lim HK, and Lim JH. Prediction of viable tumor in hepatocellular carcinoma treated with transcatheter arterial chemoembolization: Usefulness of attenuation value measurement at quadruple-phase helical computed tomography. *J Comput Assist Tomogr* 2007; **31**(2): 198–203.

17. Buckwalter KA, Ellis JH, Baker DE, Borello JA, and Glazer GM. Pitfall in MR imaging of lymphadenopathy after lymphangiography. *Radiology* 1986; **161**: 831–2.

18. Kubota K, Hisa N, Nishikawa T, *et al.* Evaluation of hepatocellular carcinoma after treatment with transcatheter arterial chemoembolization: Comparison of Lipiodol-CT, power Doppler sonography, and dynamic MRI. *Abdom Imaging* 2001; **26**(2): 184–90.

19. Willatt JM, Hussain HK, Adusumilli S, and Marrero JA. MR imaging of hepatocellular carcinoma in the cirrhotic liver: Challenges and controversies. *Radiology* 2008; **247**: 311–30.

9

Radiological diagnosis of cholangiocarcinoma

Hero K. Hussain and Isaac R. Francis

Cholangiocarcinomas are tumors that arise from the bile duct epithelium anywhere from the liver to the ampulla of Vater [1]. Intrahepatic cholangiocarcinoma accounts for 5–30% of all primary malignant hepatic tumors, and is the second most common primary malignant tumor of the liver after hepatocellular carcinoma (HCC) [1,2]. More than 90% of cholangiocarcinomas are adenocarcinomas. Other tumor types have been described. The histological grade of tumors varies from well-differentiated to undifferentiated [3]. Most tumors consist of clusters of cells, surrounded by desmoplastic stroma, which can be extensive. The latter feature makes it difficult to distinguish between reactive tissue and well-differentiated cholangiocarcinoma [3,4]. Furthermore, intrahepatic cholangiocarcinoma may be confused with metastatic scirrhous carcinoma on liver biopsy [5]. Therefore, a primary adenocarcinoma as a source for metastases should be excluded when considering an intrahepatic cholangiocarcinoma [6,7,8,9].

Cholangiocarcinoma is more common in men than women, occurring most frequently between the sixth and seventh decades [1,10,11,12,13,14]. Most patients have no predisposing risk factors, but primary sclerosing cholangitis (PSC) (5–15% lifetime risk), choledochal cysts (5% will transform and risk increases with age), Caroli's disease (7% lifetime risk), hepatolithiasis, chronic intraductal stones, bile duct adenoma, biliary papillomatosis, *Clonorchis sinensis* infection, and Thorotrast (thorium dioxide) exposure [6,12,15,16,17] are some of the risk factors for cholangiocarcinoma. A higher prevalence of positive anti-hepatitis C virus has also been associated with cholangiocarcinoma [18,19].

Anatomically, cholangiocarcinoma is classified into three broad groups: 1) intrahepatic (peripheral); 2) perihilar, which includes hilar or Klatskin tumor (at the bifurcation of the common hepatic duct [CHD]) and hepatic duct tumor (involves a major hepatic duct near the liver hilum); and 3) distal extrahepatic [3,20,21].

Primary Carcinomas of the Liver, ed. Hero K. Hussain and Isaac R. Francis. Published by Cambridge University Press. © Cambridge University Press 2010.

Intrahepatic cholangiocarcinoma arises from small, intrahepatic bile duct branches and invades adjacent liver parenchyma [2,3,6,10,12,22]. Perihilar cholangiocarcinoma or Klatskin tumor is the most common type and accounts for 50–60% of tumors. The distal extrahepatic type includes tumors that arise from extrahepatic ducts from the level of the upper border of the pancreas to the ampulla of Vater [11,15]. Fewer than 10% of patients have multifocal or diffuse involvement of the biliary tree [3,6,12].

Macroscopically, three types of cholangiocarcinoma growth have been described [23,24]: 1) the mass-forming (exophytic) type, which results in a definite mass in the liver parenchyma; (2) the infiltrating (periductal) type, which extends longitudinally along the bile duct and is either nodular or diffusely infiltrating [15]; and (3) the polypoidal (intraductal) growth type, which proliferates toward the lumen of the bile duct in the form of papillae or tumor thrombus.

Intrahepatic cholangiocarcinomas are typically mass forming and perihilar, and extrahepatic cholangiocarcinomas are mostly infiltrating; any of the cholangiocarcinomas may rarely have a polypoidal growth pattern. Combined cholangiocarcinoma encompasses more than one growth type, and is more commonly seen with intrahepatic tumors [24].

Computed tomography

Peripheral intrahepatic cholangiocarcinoma

This tumor is also referred to as "mass-forming intrahepatic cholangiocarcinoma" and is the most common type of intrahepatic cholangiocarcinoma [25]. On computed tomography (CT), they are seen as large, lobulated, intrahepatic masses, with central low density and may show mild, peripheral rim enhancement on arterial and portal venous phases of imaging with helical CT [25]. The central portion of the tumor usually is low attenuation with some areas of high attenuation. In a study of 34 tumors, 23 showed peripheral enhancement in both arterial and portal venous phase [25] (Figure 9.1) The central low attenuation areas may show contrast retention on delayed phase of imaging (usually beyond 10 minutes) [26] (Figure 9.2). In a study by Valls *et al.* of 24 patients with 25 tumors, 14 of 20 patients (70%) who underwent delayed imaging demonstrated this feature [27]. The contrast retention has been attributed to central fibrosis within these tumors. Additional findings, such as capsular retraction adjacent to the tumor and dilatation of adjacent intrahepatic bile ducts, may also be present in a small percentage of tumors [25,26,27,

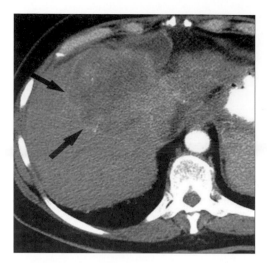

Figure 9.1 Contrast-enhanced image shows large tumor demonstrating peripheral rim enhancement (*arrows*) in arterial phase of imaging.

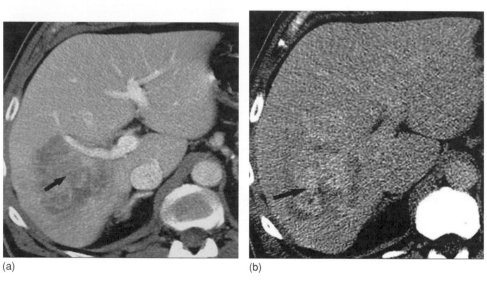

(a)   (b)

Figure 9.2 (a–b): Images obtained in portal venous phase (a) and delayed phase (b). Note tumor in posterior segment of right hepatic lobe showing contrast retention in delayed phase (b, *arrow*).

28]. In the study by Valls *et al.*, intrahepatic biliary dilatation was seen in 52% and capsular retraction in 36% [27] (Figure 9.3).

Hilar intrahepatic cholangiocarcinoma (Klatskin tumor)

These account for approximately 50% of bile duct malignancies. Infiltrating hilar tumors account for 70% of hilar cholangiocarcinomas and are seen as areas of focal

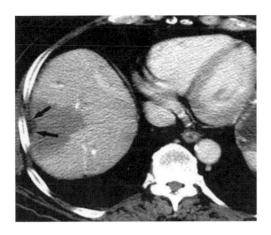

Figure 9.3 Tumor in anterior segment of right hepatic lobe. Portal venous phase shows capsular retraction (*arrows*).

eccentric or symmetric bile duct wall thickening. These tumors can be at times difficult to identify on CT, ultrasound, or magnetic resonance imaging (MRI) and may be seen as non-union of the dilated right and left ducts due to a soft tissue mass at the portal hilum (Figure 9.4, a–c). These tumors, due to their abundant fibrous stroma, tend to show hyperattenuation on delayed CT imaging [28,29]. Other types of intrahepatic cholangiocarcinoma are the 1) intraductal polypoid [30] and 2) exophytic hilar types [28,29].

Extrahepatic cholangiocarcinoma

Infiltrating extrahepatic cholangiocarcinoma is the most common type involving the extrahepatic ducts. It is usually seen as an area of focal bile duct wall thickening or a high-attenuation mass [28]. Rarely it presents as an intraluminal polypoid mass and is seen as a low-density mass within a dilated bile duct [29]. As this type of tumor tends to spread superficially, true length of involvement can be difficult to assess on cross-sectional imaging. Therefore, choledochoscopy and biopsy are often used to assess the true extent of the tumor.

Ultrasound

Ultrasound is excellent in detecting bile duct dilatation (Figure 9.5a–b) but, during the early years, it was not accurate in detecting cholangiocarcinoma. Using modern imaging equipment, the sensitivity and specificity of ultrasound in the diagnosis of Klatskin tumors has vastly improved [31,32]. Intravenous contrast agents now also allow additional improved imaging of cholangiocarcinomas [33].

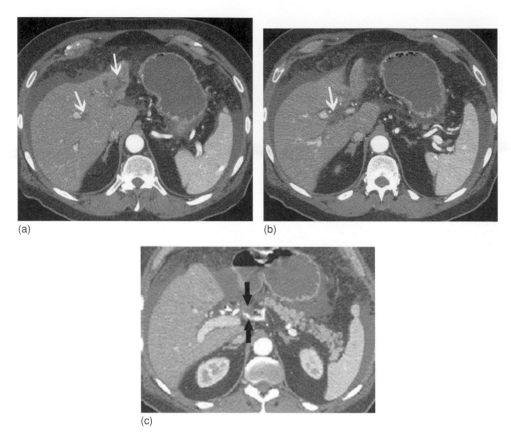

(a)

(b)

(c)

Figure 9.4 (a–c): Intrahepatic bile-duct dilatation (a–b, *arrows*) due to central mass in portal hilum. Soft tissue mass also encases hepatic artery (c, *arrow*).

Typical findings of Klatskin tumors are segmental, intrahepatic, bile-duct dilatation and non-union of the right and left ducts at the porta hepatis. Dilated intrahepatic ducts with a normal size extrahepatic duct may also be suggestive of Klatskin tumors [34,35,36,37]. Papillary tumors can be seen as polypoid masses. Despite the advances of ultrasound, it is infrequently used in most centers in the United States for the staging of cholangiocarcinoma.

Computed tomography techniques and accuracy for detection and staging of hilar cholangiocarcinoma (Klatskin tumor)

Multiphase imaging with multidetector CT (MDCT) has improved both the detection and staging of cholangiocarcinoma. Most centers use a multiphasic contrast enhancement technique consisting of an arterial phase, which is useful for arterial

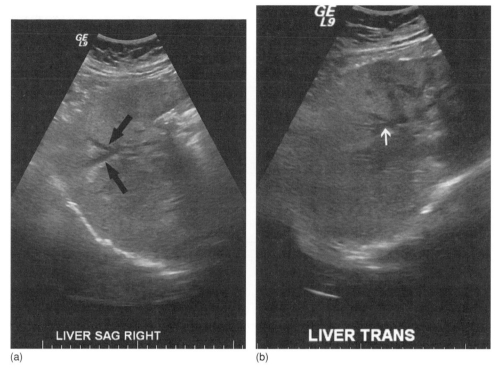

(a)   (b)

Figure 9.5 (a–b): Intrahepatic bile-duct dilatation (*arrows*) leading to portal hilum. The cause for this is poorly seen.

mapping and assessing arterial encasement; a portal venous (hepatic parenchymal) phase useful for detection of portal vein involvement; and a delayed phase at a time point of equal to or greater than 10 minutes to demonstrate the delayed contrast retention, a feature that some of these tumors may exhibit. Images can be displayed by various techniques such as multiplanar imaging and maximum and minimum intensity projection (Min IP) images of the biliary and vascular system, with the aim of displaying the relationships of the tumor and the involved vascular and biliary structures [14,38] (Figure 9.6, a–c). Such displays are useful for surgical planning prior to tumor resection as well as for radiation therapy.

The accuracy for the detection of cholangiocarcinoma using conventional CT has been reported to be between 40 and 63% [39,40], and has been improved with the use of MDCT, with some series reporting 100% detection rates [41]. The overall accuracy for predicting resectability has also improved from 40 to 60% for conventional CT to as high as 74.5% with MDCT [42]. Biliary ductal involvement is often underestimated on CT unless the results are combined with cholangiography, as

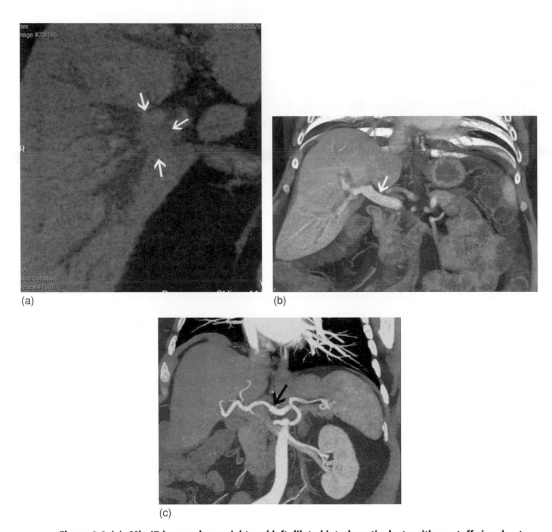

Figure 9.6 (a): Min IP image shows right and left dilated intrahepatic ducts with a cutoff sign due to central mass representing a hilar cholangiocarcinoma (*white arrows*). (b–c): Volume rendered images show patent portal vein (b, *white arrow*) and hepatic artery (c, *black arrow*).

shown in the study by Lee *et al.* [42]. In that study of 55 patients, arterial and portal vein invasion were accurately predicted by CT and cholangiography in 92.7% and 85.5% of patients [35]. In another recent study, the performance of MRI combined with magnetic resonance cholangiopancreatography (MRCP) was compared to MDCT with direct cholangiography in 27 patients with cholangiocarcinoma. Tumor extent and resectability status were assessed by two readers and were found to be equivalent for both techniques [43].

Limitations of MDCT detection and staging currently include underestimation of tumor extension and involvement of biliary tree, detection of small metastatic deposits to the liver and peritoneum, and metastases to normal sized lymph nodes [44].

A recent study compared the diagnostic accuracy of MDCT and MR cholangiography in assessing biliary ductal involvement in hilar cholangiocarcinoma and found that both techniques were equivalent: 64.3% versus 71.4%, respectively [45].

CT has limited sensitivity in assessing for nodal and peritoneal metastases, with only approximately 50% sensitivity for N2 metastases (nodal metastases to celiac axis, superior mesenteric artery, or peripancreatic, periportal, or periduodenal nodes) [42].

Magnetic resonance imaging

Gadolinium-enhanced MRI with MRCP is another comprehensive modality used for the diagnosis of cholangiocarcinoma, determination of resectability, and preoperative staging of potentially resectable tumor [6]. It provides information regarding liver and biliary anatomy, local extent of tumor, extent of duct involvement by tumor, degree of vascular involvement, and presence of lymph-node enlargement, liver metastases, and adjacent organ invasion.

Intrahepatic cholangiocarcinoma presents as a large, solitary liver mass (Figure 9.7), usually between 1 and 14 cm in diameter, with irregular, lobulated, or smooth margins [10,16,46,47,48,49,50,51]. It does not typically cause biliary obstruction [50], but satellite lesions can be seen due to its late presentation. *Perihilar and extrahepatic cholangiocarcinomas* most commonly demonstrate a nodular or diffusely infiltrating periductal growth pattern (Figure 9.8), which appears as moderate, irregular thickening of the bile duct wall (>5 mm) and narrowing of the duct lumen at the level of the tumor, usually with asymmetric upstream dilatation of the intrahepatic ducts [11].

Similar signal intensity changes are seen on MRI with intrahepatic, perihilar, and extrahepatic cholangiocarcinomas (Figures 9.7 and 9.8). Relative to liver parenchyma, the tumor is typically hypointense on T1-weighted (T1W), and hyperintense on T2-weighted (T2W) imaging [9,10,11,13,16,46,47,48,50,51,52]. The degree of hyperintensity on T2W imaging is variable and ranges from mild to marked [9,13,16,46,48,50,51,52,53]. This variability is mostly due to the amount of fibrosis, necrosis, and mucin within the tumor [16]. Occasionally, tumors can be isointense to the liver on T1W and T2W imaging [9,11,16,51,52,53,54,55].

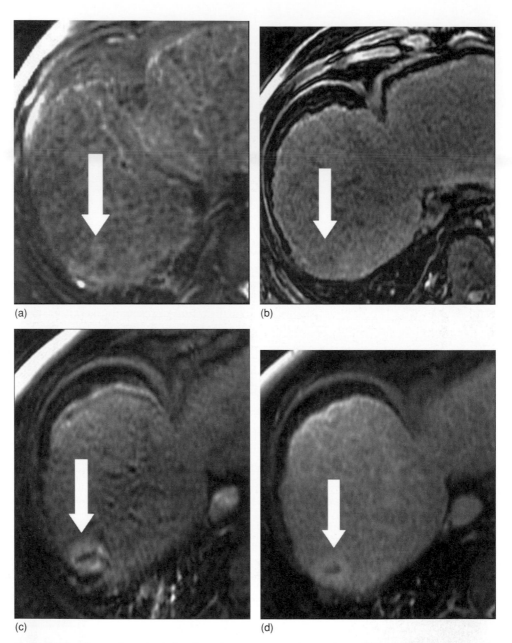

(a)

(b)

(c)

(d)

Figure 9.7 (a–d): Intrahepatic cholangiocarcinoma (*arrows*) in a patient with hepatitis C–related cirrhosis. The mass is isointense in signal relative to liver parenchyma on T2W fast spin echo (a) and precontrast fat-suppressed T1W gradient-echo imaging (b). It shows rim enhancement in the arterial phase following gadolinium injection (c), which persists in the delayed phase of enhancement (d). Because the enhancement characteristics of the mass were atypical for HCC, it was biopsied and then resected.

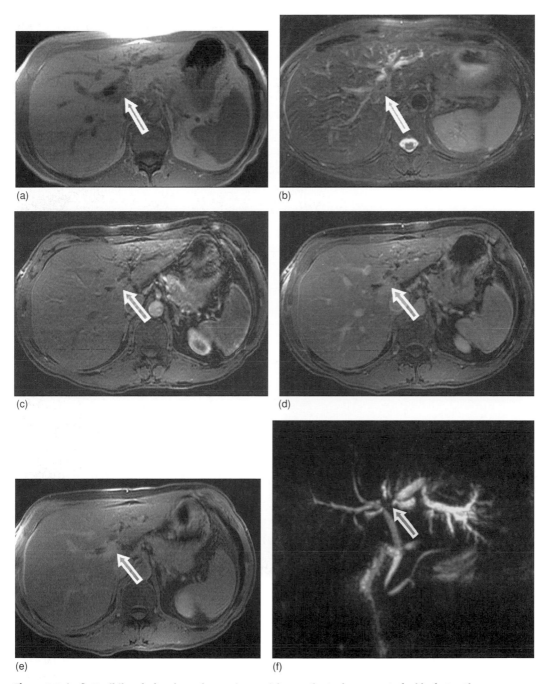

Figure 9.8 (a–f): Perihilar cholangiocarcinoma (*arrows*) in a patient who presented with obstructive jaundice. The mass is ill defined and hypointense in signal relative to liver parenchyma on T1W in-phase gradient-echo imaging (a), minimally hyperintense on T2W fast spin-echo imaging (b), enhances minimally in the arterial phase (c), and becomes more intense in the venous phase (d) but is most conspicuous on the 15-minute postgadolinium image (e). The tumor appears as a diffuse stricture on the MRCP image (f).

Cholangiocarcinoma is a hypovascular tumor. Following the intravenous administration of gadolinium chelates, the classic enhancement pattern of intrahepatic cholangiocarcinoma is heterogeneous or homogeneous with progressive and prolonged delayed enhancement [7,16,46,48,50,53,56,57]. The tumor may become isointense or mildly hyperintense compared to the surrounding liver parenchyma on delayed gadolinium-enhanced imaging [58]. Four patterns of enhancement of cholangiocarcinoma have been described on early (30 s), late (1 and 3 min), and delayed (5 min) postgadolinium imaging [16,48,49]:

1. Early peripheral enhancement with progressive and concentric filling in, which is the most common enhancement pattern;
2. Early peripheral enhancement with non-filling of the central area of the tumor (central scar);
3. Progressive and complete enhancement; and
4. Early, marked, and complete enhancement, followed by heterogeneous washout of contrast, usually from the periphery of the tumor. (This is the least common enhancement pattern.)

The variable enhancement pattern of cholangiocarcinoma is related to the amount and distribution of tumor cells and fibrous tissue in the tumor [49]. Progressive and prolonged enhancement is seen in areas of fibrosis where the blood supply is decreased and the interstitial spaces are large [48,49]. Early enhancement and late-phase peripheral washout have been shown to correspond to regions of tumor cells and reflect hypervascularity and increased perfusion.

The pattern of peripheral enhancement and delayed filling-in is not specific for cholangiocarcinoma, and a similar enhancement pattern can be seen with metastatic liver tumors [56]. Secondary signs that are more commonly associated with cholangiocarcinoma include bile-duct dilation distal to the tumor [56], segmental or lobar atrophy associated with the tumor, vascular encasement [22], central scars, and capsular retraction [7,16,46,53,59,60].

The enhancement pattern of perihilar and extrahepatic cholangiocarcinomas is similar to that of intrahepatic cholangiocarcinomas. The tumors are hypovascular and enhance slowly and gradually to a peak on delayed imaging. Because the tumors are usually smaller and typically infiltrating, they are less heterogeneous than are intrahepatic tumors. A small percentage of perihilar cholangiocarcinomas are hypervascular and enhance heterogeneously in the arterial-dominant phase [11].

Satellite nodules are less commonly seen with perihilar cholangiocarcinoma than with the intrahepatic form [11,55], probably due to the earlier presentation of perihilar tumors with biliary duct obstruction.

Perihilar and extrahepatic cholangiocarcinomas are typically seen as abnormal circumferential, extrahepatic bile-duct-wall thickening and enhancement [50,51], and are best visualized on images obtained 1 to 5 min after gadolinium administration. Duct-wall enhancement alone may not be a predictor of tumor involvement, and has been demonstrated in normal subjects [51]. It may result from fibrosis or inflammation secondary to bile-duct obstruction, and may be particularly prominent following the placement of a biliary stent [49,51]. Duct-wall thickness more than 5 mm has been suggested as a sign of tumor; however, this finding is also non-specific [51]. High-grade biliary obstruction, disproportionate to the degree of the duct-wall thickening, may be a feature of cholangiocarcinoma (Figure 9.9) [51]. Distal extrahepatic cholangiocarcinomas are frequently mistaken for adenocarcinoma of the pancreatic head [12]. Evaluation with MRCP, as with endoscopic cholangiopancreatography (ERCP), may help demonstrate the biliary origin without involvement of the pancreatic duct [12].

Associated findings

Lobar or segmental atrophy (Figure 9.10) seen in association with intrahepatic and perihilar cholangiocarcinoma [12,51,61] is thought to be secondary to tumor encasement of the portal venous branches to the tumorous lobe [16] and/or biliary obstruction [51]. Occasionally, high signal intensity on pre-gadolinium T1W images is seen in the periphery of the segments or lobes in which the tumor is present, usually around areas of duct dilatation distal to the tumor [62]. These areas show persistent increased enhancement with intravenous contrast, and are probably associated with periportal fibrosis secondary to duct dilatation.

Biliary dilatation and duct-wall enhancement are commonly seen distal to cholangiocarcinomas [51]. Sometimes there is abnormal thickening and enhancement of the duct walls, which may represent periductal tumor extension [51], or excessive fibrosis with abundant interstitial space due to cholangitis distal to the tumor [49]. In these cases, it is impossible to accurately determine the degree of periductal tumor extension. Duct-wall enhancement with or without wall thickening can also be seen in the presence of intrabiliary stents [51].

Lymph-node enlargement is common with cholangiocarcinoma, especially the perihilar type. The portacaval and porta hepatis nodes are most commonly involved

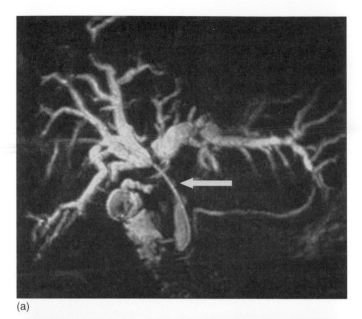

(a)

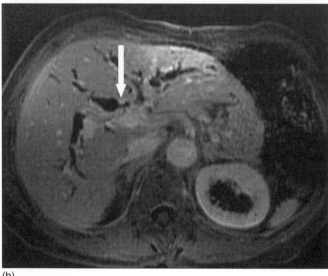

(b)

Figure 9.9 (a–b): A stent traversing a severe hilar stricture (*arrow*) on reformatted MRCP image (a). There is marked upstream ductal dilatation due to a relatively small cholangiocarcinoma seen at the level of ductal narrowing as mild thickening and enhancement of the duct wall on the gadolinium-enhanced image (b).

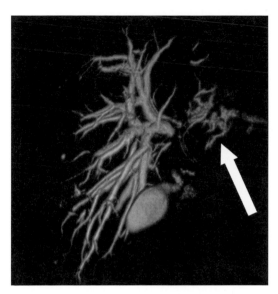

Figure 9.10 Volume-rendered MRCP image showing crowding of the left hepatic ducts (*arrow*) secondary to atrophy of the left lobe. The atrophy was secondary to obstruction of the left duct and left portal vein by a cholangiocarcinoma extending predominantly into the left lobe. (See color plate section.)

[39]. Enlarged lymph nodes are best seen on T2W (Figure 9.11) and T1W fat-suppressed, gadolinium-enhanced images [51]. Generally, a short axis diameter greater than 1 cm is used to indicate the increased likelihood of malignant involvement of the node. This criterion is neither sensitive nor specific, and we suggest reporting all visible nodes in the expected regions of metastases, regardless of their size, so that they can be examined during surgery. Intrahepatic metastases should be carefully looked for, as they may preclude surgical excision.

MRI has been shown to be useful in detecting peritoneal metastases as small as 1 cm [63,64] (Figure 9.12). Although MRI has this potential, its accuracy in detecting peritoneal metastasis from cholangiocarcinoma has not been assessed.

Vascular encasement (see next chapter) or compression can be seen with both intrahepatic and perihilar cholangiocarcinoma. Its incidence approaches 50% in hilar tumors [51,65], and it has been described in 82% of peripheral cholangiocarcinomas in a study by Soyer *et al.* [53]. Unlike HCC, it is more common for cholangiocarcinoma to encase than to invade vessels [10,66], usually the thin-walled portal veins more commonly than the hepatic arteries [22]. Encasement of the portal vein or its branches results in an autoregulatory increase in the hepatic

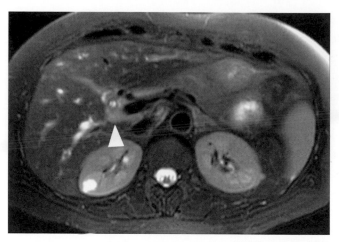

Figure 9.11 A fat-suppressed T2W fast spin-echo image showing a mildly enlarged periportal node (*arrowhead*) in a patient with hilar cholangiocarcinoma. Note that the node is slightly higher in signal relative to adjacent parenchyma on T2W imaging.

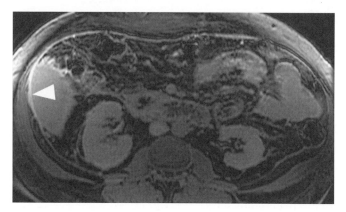

Figure 9.12 Fifteen-minute gadolinium-enhanced, fat-suppressed T1W gradient-echo image showing nodular thickening and enhancement of the peritoneum (*arrowhead*) due to peritoneal metastasis from cholangiocarcinoma. This was confirmed at laparoscopy.

arterial supply, which causes a transient increased enhancement of the affected segment or lobe in the hepatic arterial-dominant phase, also known as transient hepatic intensity difference (THID) [51,60]. Because of the tendency of cholangiocarcinoma to encase vessels, evaluation of the vasculature is necessary to assess the resectability of the tumor. Conventional angiography is considered more sensitive than MRI for detecting arterial, but not venous, involvement [9,67]. Narrowing of the vessel lumen, abrupt vessel cutoff, and focal irregular indentation are features of vascular invasion on magnetic resonance angiography [67]. The reported sensitivity and specificity of MRI for assessing involvement of the hepatic venous confluence are 75 and 98%, respectively [68].

MRCP plays an important role in the assessment of perihilar cholangiocarcinoma, and can non-invasively evaluate the biliary tree proximal and distal to an obstruction, adding accuracy to the preoperative staging [51,69,70,71]. The main advantage of MRCP over ERCP, when assessing perihilar tumors, is the ability of MRCP to evaluate suprahilar tumor extension, which is difficult to assess by ERCP because of insufficient contrast filling of ducts distal to a constricting tumor [11,13]. The main drawback of MRCP when compared to ERCP is that MRCP is solely diagnostic, whereas ERCP is also therapeutic.

Perihilar cholangiocarcinoma appears on MRCP as irregular narrowing of the bile duct involved by tumor, with asymmetric upstream dilation of the intrahepatic bile ducts. Information regarding the extent of tumor extension along the bile ducts, whether to one or both lobes, whether the tumor involves first- or second-order branches, and the presence of concomitant disease, such as hepatolithiasis [69], can be obtained from the MRCP images [13].

The reported sensitivity and specificity of MRCP compared to ERCP for the detection of bile-duct malignancy are 81 and 100% compared to 93 and 94%, respectively [61,70]. MRCP can accurately depict the presence and level of obstruction [72], and has been shown to be more effective than ERCP in delineating the anatomic extent of the cancerous infiltration [69,72].

Manfredi et al. [11] found that the level and extent of bile-duct involvement with cholangiocarcinoma using the Bismuth–Corlette classification were accurately depicted on MRCP in 83% (10 of 12) of their patients.

The combination of parenchymal and vascular information obtained from the T1W, T2W, and gadolinium-enhanced images, and bile-duct information obtained from the MRCP images, can be used to accurately stage cholangiocarcinoma. In the study by Yeh et al. [69], the authors found that MRCP was more effective than ERCP in identifying causes of the biliary obstructions and delineating the anatomical extent of the cancerous infiltration. The authors identified 84.6% (22 of 26) of cholangiocarcinomas by the presence of an enhancing mass on delayed gadolinium-enhanced MRI, obtained 5 min after gadolinium injection, but found that, in the absence of an enhancing mass, it may be difficult to characterize the etiology of a stricture [73]. Thus, MRCP images alone are inadequate for identifying the cause of biliary strictures as they provide luminal images only, and gadolinium-enhanced imaging is essential for complete evaluation of the etiology of biliary strictures.

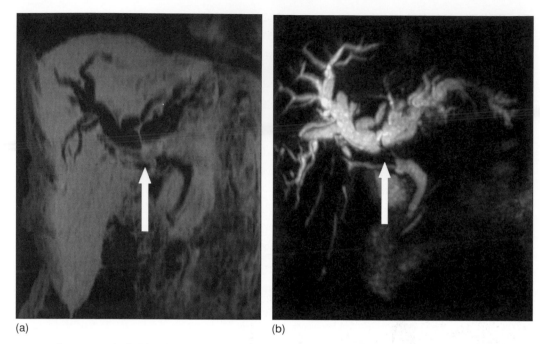

(a)   (b)

Figure 9.13 (a–b) (a): Min-IP image generated from the venous-phase three-dimensional T1W gadolinium-enhanced gradient-echo images. The ducts are of low signal on T1W images. (b): A maximum intensity projection image generated from the three-dimensional T2W fast-recovery fast spin-echo MRCP images. A hilar stricture (*arrows*) caused by a perihilar cholangiocarcinoma is well depicted on both images.

We have found that, in addition to using the standard T2W MRCP images, using the Min IP postprocessing algorithm to create projectional images of the bile ducts (Figure 9.13) from the 2-min delayed postgadolinium three-dimensional gradient-echo images is helpful for additional evaluation of the biliary tree, as this allows direct correlation of parenchymal abnormalities with bile-duct abnormalities.

Positron emission tomography

Positron emission tomography (PET) imaging has been shown to be useful for detecting peripheral cholangiocarcinoma but not specific for detecting hilar cholangiocarcinoma (Figure 9.14). False-negative results may occur with mucinous cholangiocarcinoma or may be due to the fibrous component, and false-positive results can occur in granulomatous inflammatory lesions. Fluorodeoxyglucose (FDG)-PET was found to be particularly useful in detecting metastatic disease to nodes, liver, and distant sites [74,75].

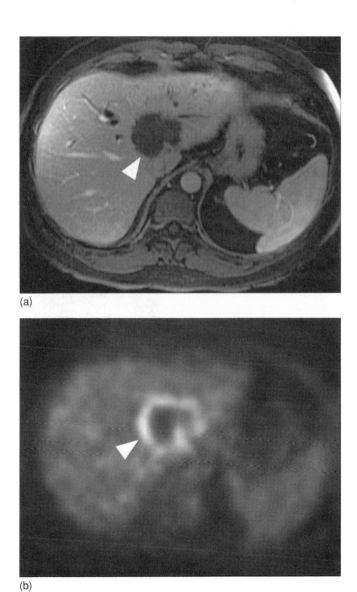

(a)

(b)

Figure 9.14 (a–b): A large, biopsy-proven periductal and intrahepatic cholangiocarcinoma (*arrowhead*) is hypovascular on venous-phase gadolinium-enhanced T1W gradient-echo imaging (a). This tumor shows uptake on FDG-PET (b).

Imaging volumetry

In patients with potentially resectable tumor, sufficient liver parenchyma should be preserved following resection to minimize postoperative liver-related morbidity and mortality. In normal livers, 25% of the total liver volume should be preserved, compared to 40% in patients with chronic liver disease or in patients who will receive preoperative chemotherapy [76,77,78].

Occasionally, the estimated remaining liver volume is smaller than required. In such cases, preoperative transcatheter embolization of the portal vein of the involved lobe is performed to redirect the portal flow to the intended non-diseased liver remnant. Redirection will induce hypertrophy of the uninvolved lobe and improve liver reserve prior to surgery [77,78].

Preoperative volumetric measurements can be acquired at CT or MRI by outlining the hepatic lobar or segmental contour on the individual slices and calculating the volumes from the surface area measurements. In this way, total liver volume as well as the volumes of the potentially resectable and remaining lobe or segments can be calculated [76].

Summary

Cholangiocarcinoma is the second most common primary liver tumor, and can arise anywhere from the small peripheral intrahepatic ducts to the ampulla of Vater. Morphologically, tumors can be mass forming or have an infiltrating diffuse or nodular periductal or intraductal growth pattern. Klatskin tumor refers to periductal tumor that involves the CHD and its bifurcation. The periductal and intraductal tumors are associated with dilatation of upstream bile ducts. The vast majority of cholangiocarcinomas have a desmoplastic stroma and show progressive delayed enhancement on contrast-enhanced CT and MRI. Ultrasound is excellent for detecting biliary ductal dilatation but not for assessing the tumor. Contrast-enhanced CT and MRI with MRCP are the imaging modalities of choice for the detection and staging of cholangiocarcinoma, with slightly higher accuracy of contrast-enhanced MRI and MRCP compared to CT. Compared to ERCP, both CT and MRI have the advantage of being able to assess the hepatic parenchyma, hepatic vasculature, and locoregional and distant metastasis, as well as the ducts, and are superior for demonstrating the distal extent of tumor, which can be difficult on ERCP due to severe ductal strictures. Underestimation of tumor extent and the inability to detect small peritoneal deposits and metastatic disease in normal-sized nodes remain the main limitations of contrast-enhanced CT and MRI. FDG-PET is useful for detecting intrahepatic cholangiocarcinoma and distant metastatic disease but not periductal tumor.

REFERENCES

1. Craig JR, Peters RL, and Edmonson HA. Tumors of the liver and intrahepatic bile ducts. In: *Armed Forces Institute of Pathology, Atlas of Tumor Pathology*, Second Series, Fascicle 26. Washington, DC: American Registry of Pathology, 1989: 197–211.

2. Ros PR, Buck JL, Goodman ZD, Ros AM, and Olmsted WW. Intrahepatic cholangiocarcinoma: Radiologic pathologic correlation. *Radiology* 1988; **167**: 689–93.

3. de Groen PC, Gores GJ, LaRusso NF, Gunderson LL, and Nagorney DM. Biliary tract cancers. *N Engl J Med* 1999; **341**(18): 1368–78.

4. Nakanuma Y, Harada K, Ishikawa A, Zen Y, and Sasaki M. Anatomic and molecular pathology of intrahepatic cholangiocarcinoma. *J Hepatobiliary Pancreat Surg* 2003; **10**(4): 265–81.

5. Rubin E and Farber J. *Pathology*, 2nd edn. Philadelphia, PA: J.B. Lippincott, 1994: 773–4.

6. Khan SA, Davidson BR, Goldin R, *et al*. British Society of Gastroenterology. Guidelines for the diagnosis and treatment of cholangiocarcinoma: Consensus document. *Gut* 2002; **51**(Suppl 6): VI1–9.

7. Maetani Y, Itoh K, Watanabe C, *et al*. MR imaging of intrahepatic cholangiocarcinoma with pathologic correlation. *AJR Am J Roentgenol* 2001; **176**(6): 1499–507.

8. Kehagias D, Metafa A, Hatziioannou A, *et al*. Comparison of CT, MRI and CT during arterial portography in the detection of malignant hepatic lesions. *Hepato-Gastroenterology* 2000; **47**(35): 1399–403.

9. Soyer P, Bluemke DA, Reichle R, *et al*. Imaging of intrahepatic cholangiocarcinoma: 2. Hilar cholangiocarcinoma. *AJR Am J Roentgenol* 1995; **165**(6): 1433–6.

10. Buetow P and Midkiff R. Primary malignant neoplasms in the adult. *MRI Clin North Am* 1997; **5**(2): 289–318.

11. Manfredi R, Masselli G, Maresca G, Brizi MG, Vecchioli A, and Marano P. MR imaging and MRCP of hilar cholangiocarcinoma. *Abdom Imaging* 2003; **28**: 319–25.

12. Jarnagin WR. Cholangiocarcinoma of the extrahepatic bile ducts. *Semin Surg Oncol* 2000; **19**: 156–76.

13. Pavone P. MR cholangiopancreatography in malignant biliary obstruction. *Semin Ultrasound CT MRI* 1999; **20**(5): 317–23.

14. Jarnagin WR, Fong Y, DeMatteo RP, *et al*. Staging, resectability, and outcome in 225 patients with hilar cholangiocarcinoma. *Ann Surg* 2001; **234**(4): 507–19.

15. Ahrendt SA, Nakeeb A, and Pitt HA. Cholangiocarcinoma. *Clin Liver Dis* 2001; **5**(1): 191–218.

16. Vilgrain V, Van Beers BE, Flejou JF, *et al.* Intrahepatic cholangiocarcinoma: MRI and pathologic correlation in 14 patients. *J Comput Assist Tomogr* 1997; **21**(1): 59–65.

17. Choi B. MRI of clonorchiasis and cholangiocarcinoma. *J Magn Reson Imaging* 1998; **8**(2): 359–66.

18. Shaib YH, El-Serag HB, Nooka AK, *et al.* Risk factors for intrahepatic and extrahepatic cholangiocarcinoma: A hospital-based case-control study. *Am J Gastroenterol* 2007; **102**(5): 1016–21.

19. Kobayashi M, Ikeda K, Saitoh S, *et al.* Incidence of primary cholangiocellular carcinoma of the liver in Japanese patients with hepatitis C virus-related cirrhosis. *Cancer* 2000; **88**(11): 2471–7.

20. Nakeeb A, Pitt HA, Sohn TA, *et al.* Cholangiocarcinoma. A spectrum of intrahepatic, perihilar, and distal tumors. *Ann Surg* 1996; **224**(4): 463–73.

21. Klatskin G. Adenocarcinoma of the hepatic duct at its bifurcation within the porta hepatis. An unusual tumor with distinctive clinical and pathological features. *Am J Med* 1965; **38**: 241–56.

22. Levy AD. Malignant liver tumors. *Clin Liver Dis* 2002; **6**(1): 147–64.

23. Yamasaki S. Intrahepatic cholangiocarcinoma: Macroscopic type and stage classification. *J Hepatobiliary Pancreat Surg* 2003; **12**(4): 288–91.

24. Lee WJ, Lim HK, Jang KM, *et al.* Radiologic spectrum of cholangiocarcinoma: Emphasis on unusual manifestations and differential diagnoses. *RadioGraphics* 2001; **21**: S97–116.

25. Kim TK, Choi BI, Han JK, *et al.* Peripheral cholangiocarcinoma of the liver: Two-phase spiral CT findings. *Radiology* 1997; **204**: 539–43.

26. Lacomis JM, Baron RL, Oliver JH III, *et al.* Cholangiocarcinoma: Delayed CT contrast enhancement patterns. *Radiology* 1997; **203**: 98–104.

27. Valls C, Guma A, Puig I, *et al.* Intrahepatic peripheral cholangiocarcinoma: CT evaluation. *Abdom Imaging* 2000; **25**: 490–6.

28. Han JK, Cho BI, Kim AY, *et al.* Cholangiocarcinoma: Pictorial essay of CT and cholangiographic findings. *RadioGraphics* 2002; **22**: 173–87.

29. Han JK, Choi BI, Kim TK, Kim SW, Han MC, and Yeon KM. Hilar cholangiocarcinoma: Thin-section spiral CT findings with cholangiographic correlation. *RadioGraphics* 1997; **17**: 1475–85.

30. Lee JW, Han JK, Kim TK, *et al.* CT features of intraductal intrahepatic cholangiocarcinoma. *AJR Am J Roentgenol* 2000; **175**: 721–5.

31. Honickman SP, Mueller PR, Wittenberg J, *et al.* Ultrasound in obstructive jaundice: Prospective evaluation of site and cause. *Radiology* 1983; **147**: 511–15.

32. Robledo R, Avertano M, and Prieto M. Extrahepatic biliary ductal cancer. *Radiology* 1996; **198**: 869–79.

33. Xu HX, Lu MD, Liu GJ, *et al.* Imaging of peripheral cholangiocarcinoma with low-mechanical index contrast-enhanced sonography and Sono Vue: Initial experience. *J Ultrasound Med* 2006; **25**(1): 23–33.

34. Meyer D and Weinstein BJ. Klatskin tumors of the bile ducts: Sonographic appearances. *Radiology* 1983; **148**: 803.

35. Yeung EY, McCarthy P, Gompertz RH, *et al.* The ultrasonographic appearances of hilar cholangiocarcinoma (Klatskin tumors). *Br J Radiol* 1988; **61**: 991–5.

36. Hann LE, Greatrex KV, Bach AM, Fong Y, and Blumgart LH. Cholangiocarcinoma at the hepatic hilus: Sonographic findings. *AJR Am J Roentgenol* 1997; **168**: 985–9.

37. Bloom CM, Langer B, and Wilson SR. Role of US in the detection, characterization, and staging of cholangiocarcinoma. *Radiographics* 1999; **19**: 1199–218.

38. Endo I, Shimada H, Sugita M, *et al.* Role of three-dimensional imaging in operative planning for hilar cholangiocarcinoma. *Surgery* 2007; **142**(5): 666–75.

39. Choi YH, Lee JM, Lee JY, *et al.* Biliary malignancy: Value of arterial, pancreatic and hepatic phase imaging with multidetector-row computed tomography. *J Comput Assist Tomogr* 2008; **32**(3): 362–8.

40. Choi BI, Lee JH, Han MC, *et al.* Hilar cholangiography: Comparative study with sonography and CT. *Radiology* 1989; **172**: 689–92.

41. Tillich M, Mischinger HJ, Preisegger KH, *et al.* Multiphasic helical CT in diagnosis and staging of hilar cholangiocarcinoma. *Am J Radiol* 1998; **171**: 651–8.

42. Lee HY, Kim SH, Lee JM, *et al.* Preoperative assessment of respectability of hepatic hilar cholangiocarcinoma: Combined CT and cholangiography with revised criteria. *Radiology* 2006; **23**(1): 113–21.

43. Park HS, Lee JM, Choi JY, *et al.* Preoperative evaluation of bile duct cancer: MRI combined with MR cholangiopancreatography versus MDCT with direct cholangiography. *Am J Radiol* 2008; **190**: 396–405.

44. Cha JH, Han JK, Kim TK, *et al.* Preoperative evaluation of Klatskin tumour: Accuracy of spiral CE in determining vascular invasion as a sign of unresectability. *Abdom Imaging* 2000; **25**: 500–7.

45. Cho ES, Park MS, Yu JS, Kim MJ, and Kim KW. Biliary ductal involvement of hilar cholangiocarcinoma: Multidetector computed tomography versus magnetic resonance cholangiography. *J Comput Assist Tomogr* 2007: **31**(1): 72–8.

46. Hamrick-Turner J, Abbitt PL, and Ros PR. Intrahepatic cholangiocarcinoma: MR appearance. *AJR Am J Roentgenol* 1992; **158**(1): 77–9.

47. Soyer P, Bluemke DA, Reichle R, *et al.* Imaging of intrahepatic cholangiocarcinoma: 1. Peripheral cholangiocarcinoma. *AJR Am J Roentgenol* 1995; **165**: 1427–31.

48. Zhang Y. Intrahepatic peripheral cholangiocarcinoma: Comparison of dynamic CT and dynamic MRI. *J Comput Assist Tomogr* 1999; **23**(5): 670–7.

49. Murakami T, Nakamura H, Tsuda K, *et al.* Contrast enhanced MR imaging of intrahepatic cholangiocarcinoma: Pathologic correlation study. *J Magn Reson Imaging* 1995; **5**(2): 165–70.

50. Low RN. MR imaging of the liver using gadolinium chelates. *Magn Reson Imaging Clin North Am* 2001; **9**(4): 717–43.

51. Worawattanakul S, Semelka RC, Noone TC, Calvo BF, Kelekis NL, and Woosley JT. Cholangiocarcinoma: Spectrum of appearances on MR images using current techniques. *Magn Reson Imaging* 1998; **16**(9): 993–1003.

52. Greco A, Stipa F, Huguet C, Gavelli A, Chieco PA, and McNamara MT. Early MR follow-up of partial hepatectomy. *J Comput Assist Tomogr* 1993; **17**(2): 277–82.

53. Soyer P, Bluemke DA, Sibert A, and Laissy JP. MR imaging of intrahepatic cholangiocarcinoma. *Abdom Imaging* 1995; **20**(2): 126–30.

54. Dooms GC, Kerlan RK Jr., Hricak H, Wall SD, and Margulis AR. Cholangiocarcinoma: Imaging by MR. *Radiology* 1986; **159**: 89–94.

55. Guthrie JA, Ward J, and Robinson PJ. Hilar cholangiocarcinomas: T2-weighted spin-echo and gadolinium-enhanced FLASH MR imaging. *Radiology* 1996; **201**(2): 347–51.

56. Awaya H. Differential diagnosis of hepatic tumors with delayed enhancement at gadolinium-enhanced MRI: A pictorial essay. *Clin Imaging* 1998; **22**: 180–7.

57. Gabata T, Matsui O, Kadoya M, *et al.* Delayed MR imaging of the liver: Correlation of delayed enhancement of hepatic tumors and pathologic appearance. *Abdom Imaging* 1998; **23**(3): 309–13.

58. Peterson MS, Murakami T, and Baron RL. MR imaging patterns of gadolinium retention within liver neoplasms. *Abdom Imaging* 1998; **23**(6): 592–9.

59. Fan ZM, Yamashita Y, Harada M, *et al.* Intrahepatic cholangiocarcinoma: Spin-echo and contrast-enhanced dynamic MR imaging. *AJR Am J Roentgenol* 1993; **161**(2): 313–7.

60. Yamashita Y. Parenchymal changes of the liver in cholangiocarcinoma: CT evaluation. *Gastrointest Radiol* 1992; **17**: 161–6.

61. Szklaruk J, Tamm E, and Charnsangavej C. Preoperative imaging of biliary tract cancers. *Surg Oncol Clin North Am* 2002; **11**(4): 865–76.

62. Yoshimitsu K, Honda H, Kaneko K, *et al.* MR signal intensity changes in hepatic parenchyma with ductal dilation caused by intrahepatic cholangiocarcinoma. *J Magn Reson Imaging* 1997; **7**(1): 136–41.

63. Low RN and Sigeti JS. MR imaging of peritoneal disease: Comparison of contrast-enhanced fast multiplanar spoiled gradient recalled and spin-echo imaging. *AJR Am J Roentgenol* 1994; **163**(5): 1131–40.

64. Low RN, Barone RM, Lacey C, Sigeti JS, Alzate GD, and Sebrechts CP. Peritoneal tumor: MR imaging with dilute oral barium and intravenous gadolinium-containing contrast agents compared with unenhanced MR imaging and CT. *Radiology* 1997; **204**(2): 513–20.

65. Itai Y, Ohtomo K, Kokubo T, *et al.* CT of hepatic masses: Significance of prolonged and delayed enhancement. *AJR Am J Roentgenol* 1986; **146**: 729–33.

66. Fernandez M and Redyanly RD. Primary hepatic malignant neoplasms. *Radiol Clin North Am* 1998; **36**(2): 333–48.

67. Lee MG, Park KB, Shin YM, *et al.* Preoperative evaluation of hilar cholangiocarcinoma with contrast-enhanced three dimensional fast imaging with steady-state precession magnetic resonance angiography: Comparison with intraarterial digital subtraction angiography. *World J Surg* 2003; **27**(3): 278–83.

68. Hann LE, Schwartz LH, Panicek DM, Bach AM, Fong Y, and Blumgart LH. Tumor involvement in hepatic veins: Comparison of MR imaging and US for preoperative assessment. *Radiology* 1998; **206**(3): 651–6.

69. Yeh TS, Jan YY, Tseng JH, *et al.* Malignant perihilar biliary obstruction: Magnetic resonance cholangiopancreatographic findings. *Am J Gastroenterol* 2000; **95**(2): 432–40.

70. Reinhold C and Bret PM. Current status of MR cholangiopancreatography. *AJR Am J Roentgenol* 1996; **166**: 1285–95.

71. Fulcher AS and Turner MA. HASTE MR cholangiography in the evaluation of hilar cholangiocarcinoma. *AJR Am J Roentgenol* 1997; **169**(6): 1501–5.

72. Lee SS, Kim MH, Lee SK, *et al.* MR cholangiography versus cholangioscopy for evaluation of longitudinal extension of hilar cholangiocarcinoma. *Gastrointest Endosc* 2002; **56**(1): 25–32.

73. Thng C, Tan A, Chung Y, Chow P, and Ooi L. Clinical applications of MR cholangiopancreatography. *Ann Acad Med Singapore* 2003; **32**(4): 536–41.

74. Kim YJ, Yun M, Lee WJ, Kim KS, and Lee JD. Usefulness of 18F-FDG PET in intrahepatic cholangiocarcinoma. *Eur J Nucl Med Mol Imaging* 2003; **30**: 1467–72.

75. Fritscher-Ravens A, Bohuslavizki KH, Broering DC, *et al.* FDG PET in the diagnosis of hilar cholangiocarcinoma. *Nucl Med Commun* 2001; **22**: 1277–85.

76. Sainani NI, Catalano OA, Holalkere NS, Zhu AX, Hahn PF, and Sahani DV. Cholangiocarcinoma: Current and novel imaging techniques. *Radiographics* 2008; **28**: 1263–87.

77. Madoff DC, Hicks ME, Abdalla EK, Morris JS, and Vauthey JN. Portal vein embolization with polyvinyl alcohol particles and coils in preparation of major liver resection for hepatobiliary malignancy: Safety and effectiveness – study in 26 patients. *Radiology* 2003; **227**: 251–60.

78. Kubota K, Makuuch M, Kusaka K, *et al.* Measurement of liver volume and hepatic functional reserve as a guide to decision-making in resectional surgery for hepatic tumors. *Hepatology* 1997; **26**: 1176–81.

10

Staging of cholangiocarcinoma

Hero K. Hussain and James A. Knol

The goal of diagnostic staging of cholangiocarcinoma is to evaluate resectability and extent of surgery, because surgery is the only curative therapy [1,2]. Cure and long-term survival can be achieved if the tumor is completely excised and the histologic margins are negative.

Staging of mass-forming *intrahepatic cholangiocarcinoma* is performed using contrast-enhanced MRI or CT. The extent and number of tumor nodules, associated portal vein narrowing or occlusion, and the presence of lymph node and distant metastasis are important determinants of survival after surgery [3,4].

Extrahepatic cholangiocarcinoma is more challenging and may require more than one imaging modality for staging. Extrahepatic tumors are classified according to their anatomical location into perihilar (Klatskin) and distal tumors [5,6,7]. Perihilar cholangiocarcinoma is typically located in the extrahepatic duct proximal to the insertion of the cystic duct [8]. Distal tumors arise anywhere from below the confluence of the cystic duct with the common bile duct to the ampulla of Vater [7]. In this chapter, we focus on the staging and preoperative evaluation of extrahepatic cholangiocarcinoma.

Perihilar extrahepatic cholangiocarcinoma

The preoperative evaluation of perihilar cholangiocarcinoma must address four critical determinants of resectability [1]:

1. Extent of tumor within the biliary tree,
2. Vascular invasion,
3. Hepatic lobar atrophy, and
4. Metastatic disease

Primary Carcinomas of the Liver, ed. Hero K. Hussain and Isaac R. Francis. Published by Cambridge University Press. © Cambridge University Press 2010.

Table 10.1 TNM staging of hilar ductal biliary cancer

TNM	Extent of tumor	Stage
Tis	Carcinoma in situ	0
		(Tis, N0, M0)
T1	Duct wall	IA
		(T1, N0, M0)
T2	Beyond duct wall	IB
		(T2, N0, M0)
T3	Liver, gallbladder, pancreas, and/or unilateral	IIA
	tributaries of portal vein or hepatic artery	(T3, N0, M0)
		IIB
		(T1,2,3, N1, M0)
T4	Other adjacent organs, main portal vein or	III
	tributaries bilaterally, or common hepatic artery	(T4, any N, M0)
N0	No regional lymph-node metastasis	
N1	Regional lymph-node metastasis	
M0	No metastasis	
M1	Distant metastases	IV
		(any T, any N, M1)

In the absence of metastatic disease, the location and extent of tumor spread along the bile ducts will determine whether it can be completely excised. If there is adjacent vascular and parenchymal involvement, partial hepatectomy, occasionally with vascular reconstruction of the blood supply to the remaining liver, may be needed. Intraoperative staging can be technically difficult; therefore, preoperative radiologic staging is crucial for determining potential surgical options [1].

There is no clinical staging system available that stratifies patients according to tumor resectability and correlates with survival. The Tumor–Node–Metastasis (TNM) staging classification of the American Joint Committee on Cancer (AJCC) (Table 10.1) is based largely on pathology and predicts survival but has little applicability to preoperative staging [1,9,10]. The Bismuth–Corlette scheme classifies perihilar cholangiocarcinoma according to its site and longitudinal extension along the bile ducts and has some therapeutic and prognostic implications [11,12]. Lateral extension of tumor is defined by the T stage of the AJCC TNM.

The Bismuth–Corlette classification is as follows:

- Type I: Tumor is confined to common hepatic duct (CHD) (Figure 10.1a). This type of tumor can be treated with segmental resection of the extrahepatic bile duct and regional lymph-node dissection [13].
- Type II: Tumor of the CHD extends to the confluence of the right and left hepatic ducts and causes obstruction at the hilum with no communication between the main right and left hepatic ducts (Figure 10.1b). This tumor is treated by bile-duct resection with hepaticojejunostomy and lymph-node dissection [13, 14, 15].
- Type IIIa and IIIb: Tumors extend into the bifurcation of the right and left intrahepatic ducts, respectively (Figure 10.1c–d). The standard surgery for these tumors is hilar bile-duct resection with hemihepatectomy of the more involved lobe, including caudate lobectomy and lymph-node dissection [13,14,15].
- Type IV: Tumor involves the bifurcation of both the right and left hepatic ducts, and usually extends to the secondary and tertiary intrahepatic ducts in both lobes, causing bilateral obstruction (Figure 10.1e). These tumors have been regarded as inoperable except for liver transplantation. Due to recent advances in surgical techniques, curative surgery is sometimes attempted if the tumor extends less than 2 cm from the hilum [16]. Multifocal tumors are also in this category.

Although the Bismuth–Corlette classification helps plan the type of surgery, the surgical procedure cannot be solely determined by this classification [17]. Papillary and polypoidal tumor may have subepithelial or mucosal spread that may not be visible on imaging and seen only with choledochoscopy or at surgery, necessitating more extensive surgery than was expected from imaging alone [2].

Lateral tumor extension and soft tissue spread can be assessed using the T stage of the TNM staging system (Table 10.1) [2]. T1 tumor is confined to the bile duct. It is usually papillary or polypoidal and presents as a filling defect within the duct [18] (Figure 10.2). T2 tumor extends beyond the duct wall. It usually presents as a periductal infiltrative or nodular mass seen on imaging as duct-wall thickening and increasing enhancement (Figure 10.3). T3 tumor is locally invasive, involving the liver, gallbladder, pancreas, or ipsilateral hepatic artery or portal vein (Figure 10.4). T4 tumor is widely invasive and involves the main or both branches of the portal vein, common hepatic artery, or adjacent organs such as the colon, stomach, duodenum, or abdominal wall [2]. Vascular involvement manifests on imaging as vascular occlusion, vascular stenosis or contour deformity, tumor contact with more than 50% of the circumference of the vessel, or ipsilateral hepatic atrophy

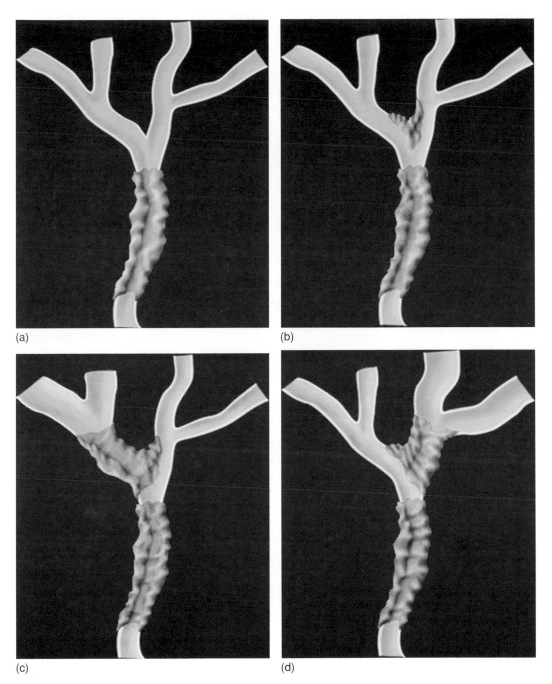

Figure 10.1 (a–e): Diagrams of the Bismuth–Corlette classification of perihilar cholangiocarcinoma.
This system classifies a perihilar tumor according to its site and longitudinal extension along the bile ducts. (a): Type I tumor confined to CHD. (b): Type II tumor involving the CHD, extending to the hilum, and obstructing both ducts with no communication between the right and left hepatic ducts. (c): Type IIIa tumor involving the CHD and the right intrahepatic duct. (d): Type IIIb tumor involving the CHD and the left intrahepatic duct. (e): Type IV tumor involving the CHD and the bifurcation of the right and left intrahepatic ducts.

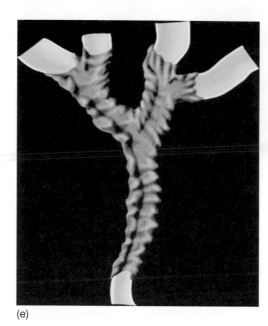

Figure 10.1 (*cont.*)

(e)

(Figure 10.4a–b) [16]. Both dynamic computed tomography (CT) and magnetic resonance imaging (MRI) are useful for assessment of vascular involvement.

The T stage of the TNM system has many disadvantages: It does not correlate with resectability [19,20,21], the distinction between stage 1 and 2 tumors can be difficult on imaging and pathology [2], and confusion between the stages can occur because of the different organs and tissues that surround various portions of the ductal systems [22]. For example, a T3 tumor of the middle extrahepatic duct which extends proximally or distally to invade the liver or pancreas is more extensive than are proximal or distal extrahepatic duct tumors invading the adjacent liver or pancreas, respectively [2].

None of these classification systems is sufficiently comprehensive. The ideal staging system should predict resectability and the need for hepatic resection, and correlate with survival [1]. Such a system will assist the surgeon in formulating a treatment plan and help the patient understand the treatment options and expected outcome. The Memorial Sloan-Kettering group has proposed a more comprehensive staging system for the T stage [1,23,24]. This classification provides the information obtained from both the Bismuth–Corlette classification and TNM staging system and is based on the extent of biliary and vascular involvement and on lobar atrophy. It also correlates with resectability and survival (Table 10.2). Using this system, researchers found that resectability was highest in the T1 group and

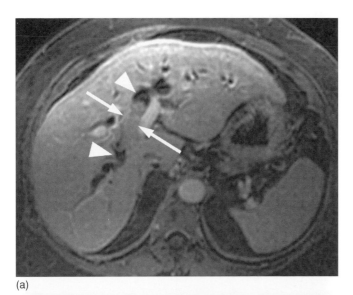

(a)

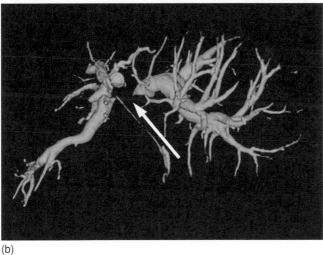

(b)

Figure 10.2 (a–b): Intraductal cholangiocarcinoma (*arrows*) at the ductal bifurcation confirmed at surgery. The tumor is seen as an enhancing intraductal mass on gadolinium-enhanced T1-weighted gradient-echo magnetic resonance image (a) and as signal loss on the volume-rendered MRCP image (b). The latter is generated from the three-dimensional MRCP series. Tumor obstructs the right and left intrahepatic bile ducts, which are dilated (*arrowheads*). There is a stent in the CHD on the MRCP image. (See color plate section.)

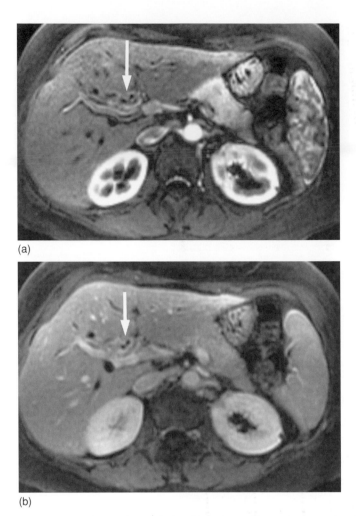

(a)

(b)

Figure 10.3 (a–f): Periductal cholangiocarcinoma (*arrows*) centered at the bifurcation of the CHD and confirmed at surgery. The tumor manifests as marked thickening of the duct wall at the bifurcation which enhances minimally in the arterial phase following gadolinium administration (a), moderately in the venous phase (90 s after gadolinium; b), and maximally at 10 min after gadolinium injection (c). The duct cutoff sign at the site of tumor is clearly seen on the minimum intensity projection image generated from the venous phase gadolinium-enhanced series (d) and on the maximum intensity projection reformatted image generated from the three-dimensional MRCP series (e). The ERCP image (f) confirms the tumor.

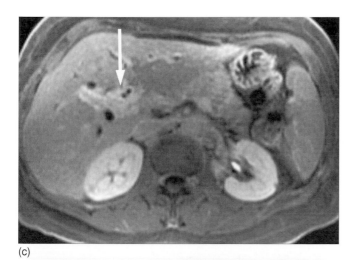

(c)

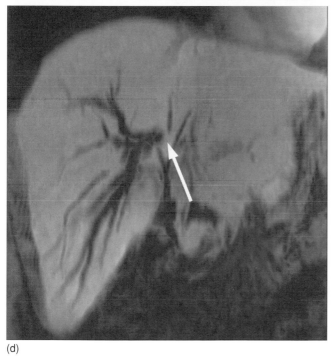

(d)

Figure 10.3 (*cont.*)

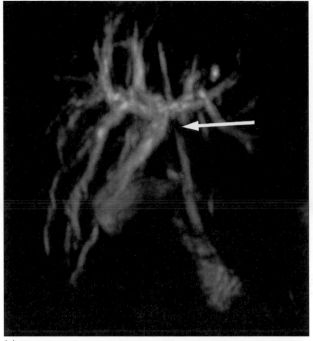

(e)

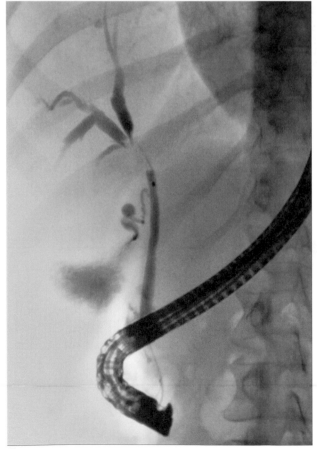

(f)

Figure 10.3 (*cont.*)

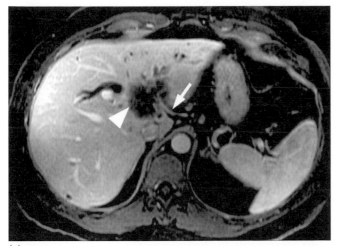

(a)

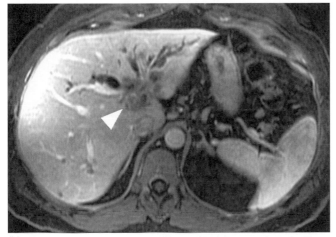

(b)

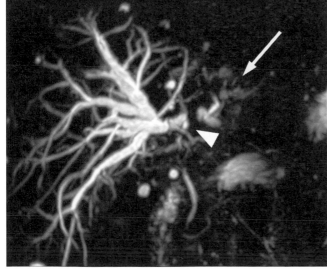

(c)

Table 10.2 Memorial Sloan-Kettering T stage for hilar cholangiocarcinoma[a]

Stage	Criteria
T1	Tumor at biliary confluence ± unilateral extension to right or left bile duct
	No ipsilateral lobar atrophy or portal vein involvement
	No main portal vein involvement
T2	T1 + ipsilateral hepatic lobe atrophy
T3	T1 + ipsilateral portal vein involvement ± ipsilateral hepatic lobe atrophy
T4	Tumor at biliary confluence
	+ bilateral extension to second-order biliary radicals
	OR + unilateral extension to second-order biliary radicals + contralateral portal vein involvement
	OR + unilateral extension to second-order biliary radicals + contralateral hepatic lobe atrophy
	OR + main portal vein involvement

[a] From [23].

decreased progressively to 0 in the T4 group. The need for partial hepatectomy for complete resection also increased with increasing T stage [23].

Staging and assessment of resectability

Currently, preoperative staging is usually performed using cross-sectional imaging modalities (CT or MRI) in combination with some form of direct cholangiography (percutaneous transhepatic cholangiography [PTC] or endoscopic retrograde cholangiopancreatography [ERCP]). Neither PTC nor ERCP alone is adequate for full assessment of tumor extent along the bile ducts [1]. PTC is considered more accurate [25,26,27]. However, the injection of contrast material through high-grade stenosis and subsequent failure of drainage may result in severe complications such as cholangitis and sepsis, and is associated with significant morbidity rates up to

Figure 10.4 (a–c): Large, masslike hilar cholangiocarcinoma (*arrowhead*) on gadolinium-enhanced T1-weighted gradient echo imaging. Tumor encases the replaced left hepatic artery (a, *arrow*), which is replaced to the left gastric artery and obstructs the left portal vein, which is not seen (b). On the minimum intensity projection MRCP image, the tumor manifests as an area of signal loss (*arrowhead*), which has resulted in atrophy of the left lobe with crowding of the left intrahepatic ducts (*arrow*). The lobar atrophy is secondary to ductal and portal venous obstruction.

7% and mortality rates up to 1% [26,28]. Compared to ERCP, magnetic resonance cholangiopancreatography (MRCP) has the advantage of showing the suprahilar ducts, which are difficult to fill during ERCP [26]. Recent advances in MRCP techniques with the development of high-spatial-resolution three-dimensional triggered T2-weighted sequences with isotropic voxel size of 1 mm enable the acquisition of high-resolution images of the bile ducts and the creation of excellent image reformats.

Cholangiocarcinoma on MRCP is seen as narrowing of or filling defects within the involved ducts. The tumor demonstrates delayed periductal enhancement on contrast-enhanced CT or MRI (Figures 10.2–10.4). Please refer to Chapter 9 for a detailed description of the imaging characteristics of cholangiocarcinoma. PTC and ERCP are useful to obtain cytologic or histologic samples, but some researchers believe that histologic confirmation of malignancy is not mandatory prior to surgical exploration and that the finding of focal biliary stenosis, together with the appropriate clinical presentation in a patient without previous surgery, is sufficient for a presumptive diagnosis of hilar cholangiocarcinoma [1].

To ensure potential survival of the patient following partial hepatectomy, there should be an adequate remaining volume of liver parenchyma to avoid postoperative liver failure. To ensure survival of the remaining liver, the remaining lobe should have an uninvolved hepatic artery, portal vein, and a first-order bile duct for anastomosis to a limb of bowel for biliary drainage. Therefore, assessment of the degree of tumor extension in the less involved lobe, the health of the remaining liver, and the search for nodal and distant metastases are crucial.

Criteria for tumor unresectability include [1,11,29,30,31]:

1. Infiltration into the second-order bile-duct branches in both lobes of the liver;
2. Involvement of major vessels including the main portal vein (>2 cm length of involvement) [16,32,33,34]), main hepatic artery, both right and left main branches of the portal vein or hepatic arteries, or involvement of the main portal vein branch in one lobe combined with involvement of the main hepatic artery in the contralateral lobe;
3. A combination of extensive vascular involvement in one lobe and bile-duct involvement to the second-order branches in the other lobe;
4. Lymph-node metastases beyond N1 station nodes; and
5. Hepatic or distant metastases.

When cholangiocarcinoma is suspected, a comprehensive search must be carried out to screen for metastatic disease. Up to 50% of patients are lymph node positive, and 10–20% have peritoneal involvement at presentation [6,35]. Nodal involvement is most common with perihilar cholangiocarcinoma, usually involving the hepatoduodenal ligament lymph nodes [36]. Regional lymph-node involvement (N1) does not make the tumor unresectable, because these nodal metastases are resected along with the primary tumor. CT and MRI are neither sensitive nor specific for the detection of metastatic nodes [2,37], and the presence of equivocal nodes cannot be used as an indication for unresectability.

Distant metastasis is adequately assessed with CT, MRI, or fluorodeoxyglucose-positron emission tomography (FDG-PET). The latter is extremely useful and has been shown to change management in up to 30% of patients [38]. In some centers, laparoscopy is performed to exclude peritoneal metastasis in those patients considered resectable on imaging [35].

Distal cholangiocarcinoma

These tumors comprise 20–30% of all cholangiocarcinomas [7,39,40,41]. Papillary tumors are more common in the distal bile duct than at the hilar region [42]. True mid-duct tumors are distinctly uncommon [7]. Distal bile-duct tumors are often mistaken for pancreatic adenocarcinoma [43]. ERCP can help determine the origin of these tumors and distinguish them from choledocholithiasis [1].

Histologic confirmation of suspected distal cholangiocarcinoma is difficult and unnecessary, unless nonoperative therapy is planned. Percutaneous biopsy of these tumors is often difficult, and endoscopic brushings have an unacceptably low sensitivity [1,44]. Complete resection is the only effective therapy for distal bile-duct tumors. Pancreaticoduodenectomy is required for complete resection [7,39,40,41,45].

Staging and assessment of resectability

Unlike for perihilar tumors, PTC is less useful than ERCP for distal tumors. MRCP is well suited to image these tumors. Similar to perihilar tumors, contrast-enhanced MRI or CT should be performed to assess extent of local extension, vascular involvement, and metastatic disease [1].

These tumors are staged using the TNM classification of the AJCC (Table 10.1). This system is of limited clinical utility because it does not take into account vascular involvement. Involvement of a short segment of main portal vein (<2 cm) does not render the tumor unresectable, because the segment of involved vein can be resected and the vein reconstructed [1]. A comprehensive evaluation of the other vessels, including the common hepatic artery and superior mesenteric artery and vein, should be conducted. Metastasis to celiac, periportal, and superior mesenteric nodes is a contraindication to surgery [39]. Lymph-node metastasis and tumor differentiation have been found to be independent predictors of outcome [7,39,41].

Diagnostic performance of imaging studies for staging cholangiocarcinoma

For estimation of the extent of biliary-duct involvement, recent studies [16,46,47] have reported an accuracy rate of 93.3% for MRI with MRCP compared to 84% for CT and PTC, but the reported accuracy for assessment of arterial and portal venous involvement is lower for MRI than for CT. Errors in staging for all modalities are often due to overestimation or underestimation of tumor extent. Underestimation may occur due to the lack of recognition of mucosal spread [26,27] or extension to the hepatoduodenal ligament [16]. Mild inflammatory changes following biliary stent placement may result in overestimation of superficial tumor spread; thus, it is recommended that all imaging be performed prior to stent placement [26,48]. CT cholangiography has also been used for evaluating the extent of ductal involvement [49].

Summary

When cholangiocarcinoma is suspected, comprehensive staging must be carried out using MRI and MRCP or contrast-enhanced CT to determine the extent of tumor spread along the bile ducts, involvement of vascular structures and adjacent organs, and the presence of metastatic disease. Imaging can overestimate or underestimate the extent of tumor in ducts and is not sensitive or specific for the detection of lymph-node metastasis. Current clinical staging systems are not comprehensive and do not help plan surgery or determine prognosis. A new comprehensive staging classification has been proposed and appears promising. Histologic confirmation is difficult and is only necessary prior to nonoperative therapy.

REFERENCES

1. Jarnagin WR. Cholangiocarcinoma of the extrahepatic bile ducts. *Semin Surg Oncol* 2000; **19**: 156–76.

2. Chung YE, Kim MJ, Park YN, Lee YH, and Choi JY. Staging of extrahepatic cholangiocarcinoma. *Eur Radiol* 2008; **18**: 2182–95.

3. Okabayashi T, Yamamoto J, Kosuge T, *et al*. A new staging system for mass-forming intrahepatic cholangiocarcinoma. Analysis of preoperative and postoperative variables. *Cancer* 2001; **92**: 2374–83.

4. Morimoto Y, Tanak Y, Ito T, *et al*. Long-term survival and prognostic factors in the surgical treatment for intrahepatic cholangiocarcinoma. *J Hepatobiliary Pancreat Surg* 2003; **10**: 432–40.

5. Khan SA, Thomas HC, Davidson BR, and Taylor-Robinson SD. Cholangiocarcinoma. *Lancet* 2005; **366**: 1303–14.

6. deGroen PC, Gores GJ, LaRusso NF, Gunderson LL, and Nagorney DM. Biliary tract cancers. *N Engl J Med* 1999; **341**: 1368–78.

7. Nakeeb A, Pitt HA, Sohn TA, *et al*. Cholangiocarcinoma. A spectrum of intrahepatic, perihilar, and distal tumors. *Ann Surg* 1996; **224**: 463–73.

8. DeOliveira ML, Cunningham SC, Cameron JL, *et al*. Cholangiocarcinoma: Thirty-one–year experience with 564 patients at a single institution. *Ann Surg* 2007; **245**: 755–62.

9. Greene FL, Page DL, Fleming ID, *et al*. eds. *AJCC Cancer Staging Manual, Sixth edn*. New York: Springer-Verlag, 2002.

10. Nishio H, Nagino M, Oda K, Ebata T, Arai T, and Nimura Y. TNM classification for perihilar cholangiocarcinoma: Comparison between 5th and 6th editions of the AJCC/UICC staging systems. *Arch Surg* 2005; **390**: 319–27.

11. Bismuth H, Nakache R, and Diamond T. Management strategies in resection for hilar cholangiocarcinoma. *Ann Surg* 1992; **215**(1): 31–8.

12. Bismuth H and Corlette MB. Intrahepatic cholangioenteric anastomosis in carcinoma of the hilus of the liver. *Surg Gynecol Obstet* 1975; **140**(2): 170–8.

13. Tsao JI, Nimura Y, Kamiya J, *et al*. Management of hilar cholangiocarcinoma: Comparison of an American and a Japanese experience. *Ann Surg* 2000; **232**: 166–74.

14. Seyama Y and Makuuch M. Current surgical treatment of bile duct cancer. *World J Gastroenterol* 2007; **13**: 1505–15.

15. van Gulik TM and Gouma DJ. Changing perspectives in the assessment of resectability of hilar cholangiocarcinoma. *Ann Surg Oncol* 2007; **14**: 1969–71.

16. Lee HY, Kim SH, Lee JM, *et al*. Preoperative assessment of resectability of hepatic hilar cholangiocarcinoma: Combined CT and cholangiography with revised criteria. *Radiology* 2006; **239**: 113–21.

17. Bold RJ and Goddnigh JE Jr. Hilar cholangiocarcinoma: Surgical and endoscopic approaches. *Surg Clin North Am* 2004; **84**: 525–42.

18. Lim JH, Jang KT, Choi D, Lee WJ, and Lim HK. Early bile duct carcinoma: Comparison of imaging features with pathologic findings. *Radiology* 2006; **238**: 542–8.

19. Hong SM, Kang GH, Lee HY, and Ro JY. Smooth muscle distribution in the extrahepatic bile duct: Histologic and immunohistochemical studies of 122 cases. *Am J Surg Pathol* 2000; **24**: 660–7.

20. Hong SM, Presley AE, Stelow EB, Frierson HF Jr., and Moskaluk CA. Reconsiderations of the histologic definitions used in the pathologic staging of extrahepatic bile duct carcinoma. *Am J Surg Pathol* 2006; **30**: 744–9.

21. Hong SM, Cho H, Moskaluk CA, and Yu E. Measurement of the invasion depth of extrahepatic bile duct carcinoma: An alternative method overcoming the current T classification problems of the AJCC staging system. *Am J Surg Pathol* 2007; **31**: 199–206.

22. Hong SM, Kim MJ, Pi DY, *et al.* Analysis of extrahepatic bile duct carcinomas according to the new American Joint Committee on Cancer Staging System focused on tumor classification problems in 222 patients. *Cancer* 2005; **104**: 802–10.

23. Burke EC, Jarnagin WR, Hochwald SN, *et al.* Hilar cholangiocarcinoma: Patterns of spread, the importance of hepatic resection for curative operation, and a presurgical clinical staging system. *Ann Surg* 1998; **228**: 385–94.

24. Sainani NI, Catalano OA, Holalkere NS, Zhu AX, Hahn PF, and Sahani DV. Cholangiocarcinoma: Current and novel imaging techniques. *RadioGraphics* 2008; **28**(5): 1263–87.

25. Otto G, Romaneehsen B, Hoppe-Lotichius M, and Bittinger F. Hilar cholangiocarcinoma: Resectability and radicality after routine diagnostic imaging. *J Hepatobiliary Pancreat Surg* 2004; **11**: 310–18.

26. Masselli G and Gualdi G. Hilar cholangiocarcinoma: MRI/MRCP in staging and treatment planning. *Abdom Imaging* 2008; **33**: 444–51.

27. Vilgrain V. Staging cholangiocarcinoma by imaging studies. *HPB* 2008; **10**: 106–9.

28. Bilbao MK, Dotter CT, Lee TG, *et al.* Complications of endoscopic retrograde cholangiopancreatography (ERCP): A study of 10,000 cases. *Gastroenterology* 1976; **70**: 314–20.

29. Szklaruk J, Tamm E, and Charnsangavej C. Preoperative imaging of biliary tract cancers. *Surg Oncol Clin North Am* 2002; **11**(4): 865–76.

30. Manfredi R, Masselli G, Maresca G, Brizi MG, Vecchioli A, and Marano P. MR imaging and MRCP of hilar cholangiocarcinoma. *Abdom Imaging* 2003; **28**: 319–25.

31. Lee SS, Kim MH, Lee SK, *et al.* MR cholangiography versus cholangioscopy for evaluation of longitudinal extension of hilar cholangiocarcinoma. *Gastrointest Endosc* 2002; **56**(1): 25–32.

32. Munoz L, Roayaie S, Maman D, *et al.* Hilar cholangiocarcinoma involving the portal vein bifurcation: Long term results after resection. *J Hepatobiliary Pancreat Surg* 2002; **9**: 237–41.

33. Neuhaus P, Jonas S, Bechstein WO, *et al.* Extended resections for hilar cholangiocarcinoma. *Ann Surg* 1999; **230**: 808–18.

34. Lall CG, Howard TJ, Skandarajah A, DeWitt JM, Aisen AM, and Sandrasegaran K. New concepts in staging and treatment of locally advanced pancreatic head cancer. *AJR Am J Roentgenol* 2007; **189**: 1044–50.

35. Khan SA, Davidson BR, Goldin R, *et al.* British Society of Gastroenterology. Guidelines for the diagnosis and treatment of cholangiocarcinoma: Consensus document. *Gut* 2002; **51**(Suppl 6): VI1–9.

36. Soyer P, Bluemke DA, Reichle R, *et al.* Imaging of intrahepatic cholangiocarcinoma: 2. *Hilar cholangiocarcinoma. AJR Am J Roentgenol* 1995; **165**(6): 1433–6.

37. Roche CJ, Hughes ML, Garvey CJ, *et al.* CT and pathologic assessment of prospective nodal staging in patients with ductal adenocarcinoma of the head of the pancreas. *AJR Am J Roentgenol* 2003; **180**: 475–80.

38. Anderson CD, Rice MH, Pinson CW, Chapman WC, Chari RS, and Delbeke D. Fluorodeoxyglucose PET imaging in the evaluation of gallbladder carcinoma and cholangiocarcinoma. *J Gastrointest Surg* 2004; **8**: 90–7.

39. Fong Y, Blumgart LH, Lin E, *et al.* Outcome of treatment for distal bile duct cancer. *Br J Surg* 1996; **83**: 1712–15.

40. Yeo CJ, Cameron Jl, Sohn TA, *et al.* Six hundred fifty consecutive pancreaticoduodenectomies in the 1990's: Pathology, complications and outcomes. *Ann Surg* 1997; **226**: 248–57.

41. Wade TP, Prasad CN, Virgo KS, and Johnson FE. Experience with distal bile duct cancers in the U.S. Veterans Affairs hospitals: 1987–1991. *J Surg Oncol* 1997; **64**: 242–5.

42. Tompkins RK, Thomas D, Wile A, and Longmire WP. Prognostic factors in bile duct carcinoma. Analysis of 96 cases. *Ann Surg* 1981; **194**: 447–57.

43. Jones BA, Langer B, Taylor BR, and Girotti M. Periampullary tumors: Which ones should be resected? *Am J Surg* 1985; **149**: 46–51.

44. Ryan ME. Cytologic brushings of ductal lesions during ERCP. *Gastrointest Endosc* 1991; **37**: 139–42.

45. Nagorney DM, Donohue JH, Farnell MB, *et al.* Outcomes after curative resections of cholangiocarcinoma. *Arch Surg* 1993; **128**: 8710–879.

46. Masselli G, Manfredi R, Vecchioli A, and Gualdi G. MR imaging and MR cholangiography in the preoperative evaluation of hilar cholangiocarcinoma: Correlation with surgical and pathologic findings. *Eur Radiol* 2008; **18**: 2213–21.

47. Park HS, Lee JM, Choi JY, *et al.* Preoperative evaluation of bile duct cancer: MRI combined with MR cholangiography versus MDCT with direct cholangiography. *AJR Am J Roentgenol* 2008; **190**: 396–405.

48. Vanderveen KA and Hussain HK. Magnetic resonance imaging of cholangiocarcinoma. *Cancer Imaging* 2004; **4**: 104–15.

49. Kim HJ, Kim AY, Hing SS, *et al.* Biliary ductal evaluation of hilar cholangiocarcinoma: Three-dimensional direct multi-detector row CT cholangiographic findings versus surgical and pathologic results – Feasibility study. *Radiology* 2006; **238**: 300–8.

Treatment of cholangiocarcinoma

11.1 Surgical treatment: resection and transplantation

James A. Knol and Shawn J. Pelletier

Cholangiocarcinoma can present anywhere along the biliary tree. Clinical presentation, preoperative evaluation, and treatment are dependent on the anatomic location of the tumor. Cholangiocarcinomas are divided into those that arise in the extrahepatic and those that arise in the intrahepatic bile ducts. Cholangiocarcinomas originating in the extrahepatic bile ducts are categorized as distal, mid, and proximal (hilar). Distal tumors are those lying in the retroduodenal and intrapancreatic bile duct. Mid bile duct tumors lie below the right and left bile-duct confluence but above the retroduodenal common bile duct. Proximal bile-duct tumors lie at or above the right–left bile-duct confluence.

Preoperative assessment

Extrahepatic cholangiocarcinoma

Patients with extrahepatic cholangiocarcinoma most frequently present with jaundice but have often had more non-specific accompanying symptoms for a few weeks to months prior to the onset of jaundice. Those additional symptoms include pruritus, mild abdominal pain, anorexia, and weight loss. Infrequently, asymptomatic patients with extrahepatic cholangiocarcinoma will be diagnosed because of an unexplained rise in serum alkaline phosphatase or bilirubin or because an imaging study done to evaluate for another condition demonstrates dilated bile ducts. The age at presentation is most frequently 60 years or greater, but younger patients, especially those with ulcerative colitis, primary sclerosing cholangitis, or choledochal cyst, may present with cholangiocarcinoma.

Initial laboratory assessment of patients with jaundice or with dilated bile ducts should include liver functions: total bilirubin, fractionated bilirubin, alkaline phosphatase, aspartate transaminase (AST), alanine transaminase (ALT), serum

Primary Carcinomas of the Liver, ed. Hero K. Hussain and Isaac R. Francis. Published by Cambridge University Press. © Cambridge University Press 2010.

albumin; complete blood count, including platelet count; prothrombin time and partial thromboplastin time; tumor markers, including carcinoembryonic antigen (CEA), cancer antigen (CA)19–9, and alpha-fetoprotein (AFP); blood urea nitrogen (BUN) and creatinine; and hepatitis serologies, including hepatitis A antibody, hepatitis B surface antigen and antibody, hepatitis B core antibodies, and hepatitis C antibody.

Imaging evaluation of the jaundiced patient is best initiated with abdominal ultrasonography, giving direction to the further evaluation of the patient. Ultrasonography will specifically look for the location and anatomic extent of any bile-duct dilation, cholelithiasis, liver masses, evidence of hepatocellular disease (cirrhosis, hepatic steatosis), and pancreatic head mass. If there are indications of bile-duct obstruction or of liver or pancreatic mass, or when there remains uncertainty of the etiology of clinical or laboratory abnormalities, additional cross-sectional imaging with computed tomography (CT) or magnetic resonance imaging (MRI) is indicated.

The too-frequent impulse to perform direct cholangiography or to achieve drainage of the obstructed biliary tree by endoscopic retrograde or percutaneous approach before more complete imaging should be avoided, because less than well-planned entry into the bile ducts will often complicate management, and may compromise staging. The only indication for biliary drainage at this point is acute cholangitis. Entering the obstructed bile duct by the endoscopic retrograde approach will necessarily result in bacterial contamination of an obstructed fluid collection, and will therefore require placement of a stent to avoid cholangitis. Percutaneous transhepatic cholangiography (PTC) of the obstructed bile duct will not usually initially contaminate the bile, but, because of a high risk of bile leak from the liver puncture site, placement of an internal or internal and external biliary drain is usually required with PTC. However, shortly thereafter, the biliary tree becomes contaminated with bacteria. For distal and mid bile-duct tumors, it has been found that, in general, there is no evidence that biliary drainage improves the management of these patients but, conversely, it has been shown to complicate their preoperative management by causing cholangitis and, in the case of percutaneous drainage, by occasional associated bleeding [1,2]. For proximal bile-duct tumors, the risks of cholangitis are multiplied by the common situation in which one side of the liver biliary tree is not drained or inadequately drained but has been contaminated through a small communication between the right and left biliary tree. In addition, the presence of a drain in the bile ducts compromises the staging of the tumor by compromising the evaluation of the longitudinal extent of the tumor proximally along the biliary tree in which the stent resides (see Chapter 10).

Imaging after initial ultrasound should begin with contrast CT of chest and abdomen and MRI with magnetic resonance cholangiopancreatography (MRCP) of the liver and pancreas, directed at both diagnosis and staging. Detailed consideration of the radiological diagnosis and staging of cholangiocarcinoma is found in Chapters 9 and 10. Staging is directed at technical resectability and tumor-related contraindications to resection, including local and distant metastatic disease. For proximal bile-duct tumors, considerations include longitudinal and lateral extent of tumor, involvement of the hilar vasculature, and the adequacy of the projected postoperative remnant liver. Resectability with respect to longitudinal and lateral extent and involvement of vasculature is discussed in Chapter 10. Because almost all resectable, proximal, bile-duct cancers will involve one primary bile-duct branch more than the other, or the vessels supplying one side of the liver, major liver resection – lobectomy or extended lobectomy (trisectionectomy) – is almost always required for curative treatment. The R0 (complete resection of tumor, negative gross and microscopic margins) resection rate and cure rates are better with concomitant liver resection for proximal bile-duct cancer [3,4,5]. In addition, for proximal cholangiocarcinoma, resection en bloc of the caudate lobe is also required [6]. Adequacy of remnant liver is usually based on the ratio of remnant liver volume to functioning liver volume, and, for normal liver, should be at least 25–30%.

Additional pertinent staging for all levels of bile-duct tumors involves evaluation for regional lymph-node metastases. Cure with positive regional nodes is unusual. Because neither CT nor MRI can distinguish benign from malignant lymphadenopathy in slightly enlarged nodes in this region, positron emission tomography (PET)-CT has been found useful, and treatment-changing information can be obtained in 16–24% of patients who were candidates for resection [7,8]. Percutaneous ultrasound- or endoscopic ultrasound (EUS)-guided biopsy is sometimes possible. Laparoscopic biopsy provides a more uniformly possible access for biopsy of suspicious lymph nodes.

Evaluation for distant metastases includes evaluation for distant nodal metastases (with CT and PET-CT) and for lung metastases (with chest CT). Non-contiguous tumor in the liver (with MRI, CT, and PET-CT) should be classified as distant metastasis – cure of extrahepatic cholangiocarcinoma with liver metastases, even when those metastases are in the projected liver resection, is essentially zero. Evaluation for peritoneal metastases (with MRI and CT) focuses on the omentum in the upper abdomen and the peritoneum adjacent to the liver and along the right abdominal wall. The presence of distant metastases is a contraindication to resection.

Pathologic proof of cancer prior to resection may not be possible with extrahepatic cholangiocarcinoma. Brush cytology can be obtained at direct cholangiography by endoscopic retrograde cholangiopancreatography (ERCP) or PTC, with sensitivity for detection of carcinoma ranging from 63 to 80%; with a triple sampling technique with brushing, forceps biopsy, and needle aspiration, sensitivity is no more than 82% and negative predictive value is low, at 39% [9]. For extrahepatic bile-duct strictures suspected to be cholangiocarcinoma, EUS with needle-aspiration cytology is diagnostic in 43–86% of bile-duct strictures at any level and in 25–83% of proximal bile-duct strictures [9]. In general, because of the infrequency of benign conditions that have a constellation of findings similar to cholangiocarcinoma [10], because of the difficulty of confirming a diagnosis pathologically preoperatively, and because of the potential loss of ability to resect a cancer after prolonged attempts at proof, most centers treating this disease will proceed to operation without pathologic confirmation of cancer [11]. Differential diagnosis of extrahepatic cholangiocarcinoma includes gallbladder carcinoma, particularly that originating in the infundibular gallbladder; primary sclerosing cholangitis; biliary sclerosis following hepatic artery chemothcrapy; Mirizzi's syndrome; postcholecystectomy focal stricture; stricture due to chronic pancreatitis; retroperitoneal fibrosis extending to the bile duct; and stone disease.

Laparoscopic staging for extrahepatic cholangiocarcinoma has only moderate usefulness when used routinely [12,13,14]. In patients with proximal bile-duct cancers considered resectable by imaging criteria, sensitivity of finding disease which at laparotomy would preclude resection is 42–65%, with most of the false negatives being due to locally advanced disease (extension along bile ducts) [12,14]. Yield for excluding patients by routine staging laparoscopy for proximal bile-duct tumor ranges from 17 to 42% [13,14]. For distal bile-duct tumors, the prevalence of peritoneal metastases is low, and laparoscopy has been found to be of no value [13].

Intrahepatic cholangiocarcinoma

Patients with intrahepatic cholangiocarcinoma present most often with a history of weight loss, increasing anorexia, and upper abdominal pain. Except when the tumor is located at the hepatic hilum and obstructs both main bile ducts, jaundice is a minor feature. Initial diagnosis of a liver mass is usually by means of abdominal ultrasonography or abdominal CT or MRI. The age at presentation is most frequently 60 years or greater. Intrahepatic cholangiocarcinoma comprises about 20–25% of primary liver malignancies, with a rising incidence.

Initial laboratory workup would be that for an unknown-origin liver mass: total bilirubin, fractionated bilirubin, alkaline phosphatase, AST, ALT, and serum albumin; complete blood count including platelet count; prothrombin time and partial thromboplastin time; CEA, CA19–9, and AFP; BUN and creatinine; and hepatitis serologies (hepatitis B surface antigen and antibody, hepatitis B core antibodies, and hepatitis C antibody).

Initial imaging is usually not able to distinguish a majority of intrahepatic cholangiocarcinomas from liver masses of other pathologies. If ultrasound is the modality identifying the intrahepatic lesion, CT of the abdomen and pelvis with oral and intravenous contrast should be done. If there is no evidence of a primary cancer within the remainder of the abdomen or pelvis, and because hypoattenuating liver lesions are most commonly metastases, a search for a primary tumor outside the liver should be undertaken: Upper and lower endoscopy, chest CT, and mammography are indicated. The radiologic diagnosis of cholangiocarcinoma is discussed in detail in Chapter 9. When the liver lesion is single, resectable, and not identifiable by other studies as a lesion not requiring resection, such as focal nodular hyperplasia or a hemangioma, preoperative needle biopsy is not indicated, because cell seeding could convert a resectable cancer to a cancer with peritoneal or body-wall implants; resection is the diagnostic procedure of choice. In contrast, with multiple nodules without evident primary tumor or when the tumor is considered unresectable or inoperable, image-guided needle biopsy is indicated.

Staging for intrahepatic cholangiocarcinoma is principally the evaluation for extrahepatic metastases: hilar and celiac lymphadenopathy, peritoneal metastasis, and lung metastasis. Suspicion of potential lymph-node metastasis, lung metastasis, and peritoneal metastasis can be strengthened by findings on fluorodeoxyglucose (FDG) PET-CT imaging, but the gold standard for eliminating resectability is biopsy. The presence of extrahepatic metastasis contraindicates liver resection for intrahepatic cholangiocarcinoma.

Preoperative treatment

Proximal extrahepatic cholangiocarcinoma

Preoperative treatment is aimed at returning the projected remnant liver to health and adequate volume to allow resection of the cancer and the surrounding liver.

Most mortality and a good portion of the morbidity after resection for proximal cholangiocarcinoma are due to liver failure. Components of that liver failure include insufficient liver volume following resection, insufficient recovery of the remnant liver from a period of biliary obstruction, and cholangitis.

Bacterbilia is commonly found at initial entry to the biliary tree obstructed from cholangiocarcinoma, but there is infrequently concomitant cholangitis. The main cause of cholangitis in the preoperative patient with cholangiocarcinoma is contamination associated with chronic biliary tube drainage combined with partial obstruction of that drainage. Because cholangitis in a portion of the liver compromises the function of the remainder of the liver, avoidance of contamination of the bile in the portion of the liver to be resected is essential. In addition, cholangitis at the time of operation is highly related to the incidence of postoperative cholangitis [4,15]. To avoid cholangitis, only obstructed bile ducts in the projected remnant liver should be entered and drained, drainage tubes should be changed at least monthly to prevent their obstruction by bile salt and proteinaceous buildup, and any cholangitis that occurs should be treated aggressively with antibiotics and assurance of drainage of infected bile. Infrequently, cholangitis occurs in the portion of the liver projected for resection despite no violation by drain placement; establishment of drainage to that portion of the biliary tree is then required.

Liver with obstructed bile ducts will atrophy, and the affected liver cells will become dysfunctional. Therefore, relief of any biliary obstruction affecting the projected remnant liver is essential, and drainage must be prolonged enough to allow return of normal liver function in that remnant liver, usually signified by the serum total bilirubin returning to normal [16]. If there appears to be adequate anatomic decompression of the biliary obstruction but bilirubin does not return to normal, either cholangitis or underlying hepatocellular disease is the likely reason. With either of these conditions, proceeding with a major liver resection is a predictor of postoperative liver failure.

Very frequently, resection of proximal cholangiocarcinoma will require an extended right or left hepatectomy. In order to achieve an adequate liver remnant to avoid postoperative liver failure, most centers are routinely using portal vein embolization of the liver lobe to be resected, causing atrophy of the embolized lobe and induced hypertrophy of the future liver remnant [17,18,19). The usual time allowed for hypertrophy after portal vein embolization prior to the operation is 1 month, but volumetrics at that point should be repeated to determine whether more time is needed to allow additional hypertrophy of the liver remnant.

Mid and distal extrahepatic cholangiocarcinoma

No preoperative treatment is usually required prior to operation for mid and distal bile-duct cancers. Biliary drainage has been found in multiple studies to increase the risk of complications in this group of patients, with no apparent benefit [1,2]. The possible exception is in patients who are severely jaundiced (bilirubin >20 mg/dL), in which case many surgeons would establish biliary drainage for a period of time before operating, although there are few data to support or contradict drainage in this markedly jaundiced group. In patients in whom biliary drainage has been established, aggressive treatment of cholangitis is required prior to operation.

Intrahepatic cholangiocarcinoma

Large intrahepatic cholangiocarcinomas will often have central necrosis, which may be associated with fever and, very infrequently, with infection. In addition, there are usually multiple obstructed small bile ducts peripheral to the tumor, and there can be associated cholangitis in these obstructed bile ducts, manifested by fever. Blood cultures should be obtained. Appropriate antibiotics should be directed against the cultured organisms for an adequate treatment course prior to resection. If cultures are negative, empiric antibiotics are indicated when the clinical picture suggests cholangitis. Where the intrahepatic cholangiocarcinoma obstructs a major bile duct, if the tumor is resectable, biliary drainage of the portion of liver to be resected should be avoided. If the patient is jaundiced, if a major bile duct draining the projected remnant liver is obstructed, that bile duct should be drained and liver function restored.

In cases where the intrahepatic cholangiocarcinoma is technically resectable but the projected liver remnant is too small, based on volumetrics, portal vein embolization of the lobe containing the tumor should be performed to induce hypertrophy in the projected remnant liver, and time be allowed (usually at least 1 month) to achieve adequate hypertrophy in the projected remnant liver before resection [17].

Operative treatment

Surgical resection is the only treatment that can potentially cure cholangiocarcinoma. The operative treatment used for cholangiocarcinoma is selected based upon the anatomic location of the tumor and the associated structures involved. In a few centers, transplantation is performed for highly selected patients with proximal extrahepatic cholangiocarcinoma.

Proximal extrahepatic bile-duct cancer

It has been found that R0 resection of proximal bile-duct cancer is more often achieved by resection of the tumor combined with an en bloc liver resection than with resection of the bile duct without liver resection [3,4,5]. The portion of liver to be resected and that to be preserved are almost always determined preoperatively, and that determination is rarely changed intraoperatively (see Chapter 10). Requirements for the remnant liver are that it has blood supply from both portal vein and artery, that it has venous drainage, that it has adequate bile drainage, and that its volume and health are enough to prevent postoperative liver failure. The resection recommended, then, is resection of the bile duct from where it approaches the pancreas up to and including the bile-duct bifurcation and enough of the bile duct on the remnant liver side to achieve a microscopically negative margin (there are data suggesting that a ≥ 5 mm margin on the bile duct is needed for best results [20]), en bloc with the gallbladder and the liver selected for resection, to include the caudate lobe [6]. The portal, retroduodenal, superior retropancreatic, hepatic artery, and celiac lymph nodes are also resected. Reconstruction of the biliary drainage uses a Roux-en-Y limb, usually brought retrocolic to the hepatic flexure. Infrequently, a segment of portal vein must be resected to remove the tumor, and the vein is reconstructed. Such portal vein resection has been found not to increase the mortality or morbidity of the procedure in some studies, but has in others, but may improve the chance of an R0 resection [21,22]. Occasionally the inferior extent of the tumor requires concomitant pancreatoduodenectomy with hepatectomy to achieve an R0 resection, but there is a significant increase in the mortality and morbidity associated with such an operation [23,24]. Resection and reconstruction of the arterial supply to the remnant liver is discouraged, based upon poor results with respect to tumor-free survival in patients requiring arterial resection [25].

Complications following resection for proximal bile-duct cholangiocarcinoma occur in 14–64% of patients and include hepatic failure, wound infection, bile leak, intraabdominal abscess, stricture at the biliary-enteric anastomosis, portal vein thrombosis, hepatic artery thrombosis, and intraabdominal bleeding [4,15,18,20,26]. Operative mortality ranges from 0 to 15% [4,15,18,20,26,27].

Adjuvant treatment for proximal bile-duct cancer is almost exclusively postoperative, and has been found beneficial, without studies available differentiating its use based upon staging. Adjuvant therapy is recommended particularly with node-positive tumors and in patients with positive margins (R1: gross resection of tumor, but with microscopic margins positive, or R2: incomplete resection of tumor, with gross margins positive) [28]. Usually adjuvant therapy is radiochemotherapy, with additional chemotherapy after the completion of the radiotherapy.

Between 35 and 70% of proximal bile-duct tumors are reported as resectable for cure; the lower percentage is more likely to be accurate due to selection taking place among patients who finally arrive at a specialty center [4,18,20,21,26]. Five-year survival following R0 resection for proximal bile-duct cancer is 37–46% [20,21,26], and median survival is 46 to 53 months [4,20,21]. Five-year survival for R1 resection is 31–35% [20,26] and for R2 resection is 0% [20]. Factors indicating a worse prognosis after resection include regional lymph-node metastases, positive surgical margins, portal vein resection, hepatic artery resection, no hepatectomy, and poorly differentiated tumor [3,4,20,22].

Mid bile-duct extrahepatic cholangiocarcinoma

Anatomically, these cancers do not involve the bile-duct confluence and do not involve the common bile duct where it enters the pancreas. Often, these tumors extend proximal or distal to these arbitrary divisions, affecting the choice of operation that is required to resect them. Resection of these tumors requires resection of the mid bile duct and gallbladder, and often may require resection of the portal vein, which then requires reconstruction. Morbidity and mortality associated with concomitant resection of the hepatic artery have been high. Because of extension to the level of the upper border of the pancreas, pancreatoduodenectomy (see distal bile-duct cancers) is often performed to achieve a negative distal margin. Less commonly, resection with combined hepatectomy is performed, and, even less commonly, combined pancreatoduodenectomy with liver resection is required [29,30,31). Portal, retroduodenal, supra- and retropancreatic, and celiac lymph-node dissection is usually performed. Reconstruction of the biliary tree is accomplished by Roux-en-Y hepaticojejunostomy.

Major complications following resection for mid bile-duct cancers occur in 12–30% of patients and include wound infection, bile leak, pancreatic leak, intraabdominal abscess, stricture at the biliary-enteric anastomosis, portal vein thrombosis, pseudoaneurysm of the adjacent vessels, and intraabdominal bleeding [29,30]. If vascular resection with reconstruction is performed, thrombosis or pseudoaneurysm involving those vessels is more common, and liver ischemia or even liver failure is possible. Operative mortality ranges from 2 to 7% [29,30,31].

Adjuvant treatment for mid bile-duct cancer has not been studied specifically. Extrapolation from other bile-duct tumors is used, and treatment is almost exclusively postoperative. Indications include lymph-node metastases, tumor extension (T>2), or positive surgical margins. Usually adjuvant therapy is radiochemotherapy, with additional chemotherapy after the completion of the radiotherapy. There exist no prospective controlled studies substantiating benefit of adjuvant therapy with these tumors.

Approximately 85% of mid bile-duct tumors are resectable, although achieving negative radial margins is challenging because of the adjacent portal vein and hepatic artery [29,30]. Radial margins in resected mid bile-duct tumors are positive (R1 or R2) in 25–50% of patients [29,31]. Five-year survival for mid bile-duct cancer following resection is 24–31% [29,31], with a median survival of 39 months [31]. Five-year survivals after R1 and R2 resections are 16 and 0%, respectively [30]. Factors indicating a worse prognosis after resection include regional lymph-node metastases, positive surgical margins, depth of tumor invasion into the bile-duct wall, and need for blood transfusions [29,30,31].

Distal extrahepatic bile-duct cholangiocarcinoma

These cancers are grouped, for purposes of operative strategy, with other peri-ampullary cancers, which also include ampulla of Vater cancer, pancreatic head cancer, and cancer of the first, second, and proximal portions of the third part of the duodenum. Frequently the exact origin of a cancer in this region cannot be determined until the region is examined by the pathologist after resection. The most commonly performed operation for these tumors is *standard pancreatoduodenectomy*, which is also known as Whipple's procedure. This operation includes en bloc resection of the distal bile duct, the pancreatic head, the distal stomach, the entire duodenum and about 15 to 20 cm of the proximal jejunum, and the adjacent and included lymph nodes. Occasionally a segment of the portal vein is resected and reconstructed. Reconstruction requires pancreatojejunostomy, hepatodochojejunostomy, and gastrojejunostomy, usually in that order, with the gastrojejunostomy usually performed as an antecolic anastomosis. Some surgeons prefer anastomosing the pancreas to the stomach. The *pylorus-sparing pancreatoduodenectomy* is an alternative operation, similar to the standard operation with the difference that the distal stomach, the pylorus, about 2 cm of the proximal duodenum, and the right gastric artery are not resected. Because the lymph nodes associated with the right gastric artery and along the right gastroepiploic artery are not as reliably taken with the pylorus-sparing operation, it may not be an appropriate cancer operation in many cases of distal bile-duct cancer. Recent studies have not indicated an advantage to the pylorus-sparing operation [32].

Complications following pancreatoduodenectomy occur in 18–35% of patients and include wound infection, intraabdominal abscess, pancreatic fistula, biliary fistula, gastric fistula, delayed gastric emptying, cardiac complications, deep venous thrombosis, pulmonary embolism, pneumonia, bleeding, and portal vein thrombosis [27,33]. Operative mortality is in the range of 3% [27,33].

Adjuvant treatment for distal bile-duct cancer is almost exclusively postoperative, and is indicated when there are regional lymph-node metastases, for pT>2 tumors, or when resection margins are positive. Usually adjuvant therapy is radiochemotherapy, with additional chemotherapy after the completion of the radiotherapy. Detailed discussion of adjuvant therapy is found in the following chapters.

Distal bile-duct tumors are resectable for cure in 43–96% of patients [27,33,34]. Survival for distal bile-duct cancer following R0 resection includes 5-year survival of 25–27% and median survival of 25 to 35 months [27,33,34]. Factors indicating a worse prognosis after resection include regional lymph-node metastases, positive surgical margins, larger tumors, poor tumor differentiation, and positive p53 expression [27,33,34].

Intrahepatic cholangiocarcinoma

Liver resection based upon the location of the tumor is the recommended treatment for these tumors. For peripherally placed tumors, hilar lymph-node resection is not generally done [35], with the presence of hilar lymph-node metastases considered a relative contraindication to resection because of a generally short survival for most patients [27,36]. For intrahepatic tumors extending to the hepatic hilum, extrahepatic bile-duct resection and lymph-node dissection, in addition to liver resection, is performed. Radiofrequency ablation has been used for treatment of additional tumors that cannot be safely included within the resection margins. There are few data regarding treatment of these tumors by radiofrequency ablation alone.

Complications following liver resection for intrahepatic cholangiocarcinoma occur in 11–38% of patients and include wound infection, ascites, pleural effusion, liver failure, intraabdominal abscess, bile leak, cardiac complications, deep venous thrombosis, pulmonary embolism, pneumonia, and bleeding [35,37,38]. Operative mortality is reported as 1.2–7% [27,35,36,37,38].

Adjuvant treatment for intrahepatic cholangiocarcinoma is almost exclusively postoperative, and has been recommended in patients with multiple tumors and/or node-positive tumors and in patients with positive margins [37], but there remain questions about effectiveness [27]. For discussion of radiotherapy and chemotherapy for these tumors, please see the subsequent chapters.

Between 32 and 75% of intrahepatic cholangiocarcinomas are resectable [27,35,37,38]. Five-year survival after resection ranges from 17 to 40% [27,35,36], and median survival is 25 to 53 months [27,36]. Five-year survival for resections with positive margins is 0–20% [27,35,36]. Factors indicating a worse prognosis after resection include multiple intrahepatic tumors, positive surgical margins, lymph-node metastases, vascular invasion, and size of the tumor [27,36,37].

Transplantation for cholangiocarcinoma

Transplantation for cholangiocarcinoma is controversial because of its use of a scarce resource, the donated liver or partial liver, for a disease that historically has had poor survival with transplantation, worse survival than that of other diseases for which the scarce livers for transplantation can be used [39,40]. Liver transplantation has been used for proximal extrahepatic cholangiocarcinoma most frequently, but has also been used for treatment of intrahepatic cholangiocarcinoma. In patients with primary sclerosing cholangitis with a known propensity for cholangiocarcinoma, indications for liver transplant have been usually based upon the level of liver dysfunction; but liver transplantation is also used in patients with primary sclerosing cholangitis who have cholangiocarcinoma, because there are no other surgical options, due to cirrhosis, portal hypertension, and tumor multicentricity. Transplant is performed both after total hepatectomy with removal of the common hepatic duct [41] and after total hepatectomy combined with pancreatoduodenectomy to remove the entire biliary system [42]. Results of transplantation alone for proximal extrahepatic cholangiocarcinoma have yielded 5-year survivals from 22 to 38% [41,43,44,45,46,47,48]; therefore, transplantation is not recommended. Similarly, transplantation for intrahepatic cholangiocarcinoma has resulted in 5-year survivals of 20–42% [49,50,51] and is thought not to justify use of a donor liver.

Table 11.1.1 Enrollment criteria for liver transplantation protocol for patients with proximal extrahepatic cholangiocarcinoma at the Mayo Clinic[a]

Diagnosis of cholangiocarcinoma

Unresectable hilar cholangiocarcinoma, or cholangiocarcinoma in patients with primary sclerosing cholangitis (excludes intrahepatic and mid and distal bile-duct cholangiocarcinoma)

Diagnosis must be made by one of:
  Brush cytology
  Intraluminal biopsy
  CA19–9 > 100 U/mL
  Biliary aneuploidy with digital imaging analysis and fluorescent in situ hybridization

Tumor characteristics

Must be unresectable as judged by an experienced hepatobiliary surgeon

Clinical staging must include CT of the chest and abdomen, liver ultrasonography, bone scan, and EUS with fine-needle aspiration of any suspicious lymph nodes

Radial dimensions of any mass lesion must be ≤3 cm

No intrahepatic or extrahepatic metastases

Exclusion criteria

Previous abdominal radiotherapy

Transperitoneal biopsy of the tumor

Prior attempt at resection with violation of the bile ducts

Uncontrolled infection

Medical condition precluding liver transplant

Other malignancy than skin or cervix within the previous 5 years

---

[a] From [53].

The Mayo Clinic has reported the only acceptable results from liver transplantation for hilar cholangiocarcinoma, with a 5-year survival of 71% of patients transplanted [52]. The experience is based on a strict protocol started in 1993, with criteria for enrollment listed in Table 11.1.1. Patients who meet criteria are treated with preoperative radiochemotherapy: external beam radiotherapy, continuous 5-fluorouracil, and brachytherapy [53]. Within 2 weeks following completion of brachytherapy, exploratory laparoscopy is performed to exclude peritoneal and lymph-node metastases. Capecitabine is continued after the radiotherapy until transplant. A recent review reported that 148 patients enrolled, and 90 (60.8%) completed the neoadjuvant therapy and transplant [52]. Thirty-nine patients (26%) were removed from candidacy because of death or progression of disease.

Factors portending a poorer prognosis for survival and recurrent disease have been increased age, pretransplant CA19–9 $\geq$ 100 U/mL, prior cholecystectomy, mass seen on cross-sectional imaging, residual tumor >2 cm in diameter in the explant, high tumor grade, and perineural invasion in the explant [54]. Factors responsible for the superior results with this protocol over the results reported by others are likely due to the strict entry criteria (Table 11.1.1 – only patients with Stage I and IIA are candidates for entry), the regimen of neoadjuvant radiochemotherapy, the exclusion of patients who have had transperitoneal aspiration or biopsy, and the pretransplant laparoscopy for exclusion of patients with peritoneal or lymph-node metastases.

Despite these excellent results, treatment for hilar cholangiocarcinoma that is amenable to resection should continue to be treated by resection; results at the Mayo Clinic must be duplicated at other institutions before wide adoption, and patients with more advanced-stage disease which is resectable should have the opportunity for effective treatment of their cancer [55]. In addition, future trials of neoadjuvant therapy, probably excluding radiotherapy, should be strongly considered.

Summary

Surgical treatment for cholangiocarcinoma is the only currently available treatment modality that is able to regularly affect cures, but surgical treatment is able to do so only in selected patients. Selection of patients with cholangiocarcinoma for resection requires preoperative assessment to exclude patients with distant metastatic cancer and with locally inoperable cancer. Determination of local operability requires preoperative evaluation of radial and longitudinal extent of the cancer and assessment of regional lymph nodes. Tumors that require liver resection as part of the operative procedure are proximal extrahepatic and intrahepatic cholangiocarcinoma. Evaluation for such resections requires that the health of the liver, optimization of function of the remnant liver, and the predicted volume of the remnant liver be determined in assessing the operability of the patient. Avoidance of and preoperative aggressive treatment of cholangitis are necessary for satisfactory results from operation. For patients requiring liver resection, adequate preoperative biliary decompression of the remnant liver and promotion of hyperplasia of the remnant liver by portal vein embolization of the liver slated for resection are vital in decreasing morbidity and mortality. The resectability of cholangiocarcinoma is greater for distal than for proximal extrahepatic or intrahepatic tumor locations. The 5-year survivals for R0 resected patients, however, are in the 20–40% range no matter where the tumor is located and despite multimodality therapy. Recently, better survivals have been reported for proximal extrahepatic cholangiocarcinomas treated by liver transplantation after neoadjuvant radiochemotherapy, but these results are in the face of highly restrictive patient selection. Nevertheless, over the past 15 years, more aggressive resections implementing liver resections, vascular reconstructions, or transplant have achieved modest improvements in operability and survival, particularly for patients with the more-difficult-to-treat proximal bile-duct cancers.

REFERENCES

1. Limongelli P, Pai M, Bansi D, *et al.* Correlation between preoperative biliary drainage, bile duct contamination and postoperative outcomes for pancreatic surgery. *Surgery* 2007; **142**: 313–18.

2. Povoski SP, Karpeh MS Jr., Conlon KC, Blumgart LH, and Brennan MF. Association of preoperative biliary drainage with postoperative outcome following pancreaticoduodenectomy. *Ann Surg* 1999; **230**: 143–4.

3. Ito F, Agni R, Rettammel MA, *et al.* Resection of hilar cholangiocarcinoma: Concomitant liver resection decreases hepatic recurrence. *Ann Surg* 2008; **248**: 273–9.

4. Jarnigan WR, Fong Y, DeMatteo RP, *et al.* Staging, resectability, and outcome in 225 patients with hilar cholangiocarcinoma. *Ann Surg* 2001; **234**: 507–19.

5. Tsao JI, Nimura Y, Karniya J, *et al.* Management of hilar cholangiocarcinoma: Comparison of an American and a Japanese experience. *Ann Surg* 2000; **232**: 166–74.

6. Kondo S, Takada T, Mayazaki M, *et al.* Guidelines for the management of biliary tract and ampullary carcinomas: Surgical treatment. *J Hepatobiliary Pancreat Surg* 2008; **15**: 41–54.

7. Kim JY, Kim MH, Lee TY, *et al.* Clinical role of 18F-FDG PET-CT in suspected and potentially operable cholangiocarcinoma: A prospective study compared with conventional imaging. *Am J Gastroenterol* 2008; **103**: 1145–51.

8. Corvera CU, Blumgart LH, Akhurst T, *et al.* 18F-fluorodeoxyglucose positron emission tomography influences management decisions in patients with biliary cancer. *J Am Coll Surg* 2008; **206**: 47–65.

9. Pavey DA and Gress FG. The role of EUS-guided FNA for the evaluation of biliary strictures. *Gastrointest Endosc* 2006; **64**: 334–7.

10. Corvera CU, Blumgart LH, Darvishian F, *et al.* Clinical and pathologic features of proximal biliary strictures masquerading as hilar cholangiocarcinoma. *J Am Coll Surg* 2005; **201**: 862–9.

11. Jarnigan WR. Cholangiocarcinoma of the extrahepatic bile ducts. *Semin Surg Oncol* 2000; **19**: 156–76.

12. Weber SM, DeMatteo RP, Fong Y, Blumgart LH, and Jarnagin WR. Staging laparoscopy in patients with extrahepatic biliary carcinoma. *Ann Surg* 2002; **235**: 392–9.

13. Vollmer CM, Drebin JA, Middleton WD, *et al.* Utility of staging laparoscopy on subsets of peripancreatic and biliary malignancies. *Ann Surg* 2002; **235**: 1–7.

14. Connor S, Barron E, Wigmore SJ, Madhavan KK, Parks RW, and Garden OJ. The utility of laparoscopic assessment in the preoperative staging of suspected hilar cholangiocarcinoma. *J Gastrointest Surg* 2005; **9**: 476–80.

15. Sano T, Shimada K, Sakamoto Y, Yamamoto J, Yamasaki S, and Kosuge T. One hundred two consecutive hepatobiliary resections for perihilar cholangiocarcinoma with zero mortality. *Ann Surg* 2006; **244**: 240–7.

16. Maguchi H, Takahashi K, Katanuma A, *et al.* Preoperative biliary drainage for hilar cholangiocarcinoma. *J Hepatobiliary Pancreat Surg* 2007; **14**: 441–6.

17. Heming AW, Reed AI, Howard RJ, *et al.* Preoperative portal vein embolization for extended hepatectomy. *Ann Surg* 2003; **237**: 686–93.

18. Kawasaki S, Imamura H, Kobayashi A, Noike T, Miwa S, and Miyagawa S. Results of surgical resection for patients with hilar bile duct cancer: Application of extended hepatectomy after biliary drainage and hemihepatic portal vein embolization. *Ann Surg* 2003; **238**: 84–92.

19. Yokoyama Y, Nagino M, Nishio H, Ebata T, Igami T, and Nimura Y. Recent advances in the treatment of hilar cholangiocarcinoma: Portal vein embolization. *J Hepatobiliary Pancreat Surg* 2007; **14**: 447–54.

20. Seyama Y, Kubota K, Sano K, *et al.* Long-term outcome of extended hemihepatectomy for hilar bile duct cancer with no mortality and high survival rate. *Ann Surg* 2003; **238**: 73–83.

21. Heming AL, Reed AI, Fujita S, Foley DP, and Howard RJ. Surgical management of hilar cholangiocarcinoma. *Ann Surg* 2005; **241**: 693–702.

22. Miyazaki M, Kato A, Ito H, *et al.* Combined vascular resection in operative resection for hilar cholangiocarcinoma: Does it work? *Surgery* 2007; **141**: 581–8.

23. Hirono S, Tani M, Kawai M, Ina S, Uchiyama K, and Yamaue H. Indication of hepatopancreatoduodenectomy for biliary tract cancer. *World J Surg* 2006; **30**: 567–73.

24. Wakai T, Shirai Y, Tsuchiya Y, Nomura T, Akazawa K, and Hatakeyama K. Combined major hepatectomy and pancreaticoduodenectomy for locally advanced biliary carcinoma: Long term results. *World J Surg* 2008; **32**: 1075–6.

25. Miyazaki M, Kimura F, Shimizu H, *et al.* Recent advance in the treatment of hilar cholangiocarcinoma: Hepatectomy with vascular resection. *J Hepatobiliary Pancreat Surg* 2007; **14**: 463–8.

26. Konstadoulakis MM, Roayaie S, Gomatos IP, *et al.* Aggressive surgical resection of hilar cholangiocarcinoma: Is it justified? Audit of a single center's experience. *Am J Surg* 2008; **196**: 160–9.

27. DeOliveira ML, Cunningham SC, Cameron JL, *et al.* Cholangiocarcinoma: Thirty-one-year experience with 564 patients at a single institution. *Ann Surg* 2007; **245**: 755–62.

28. Cheng Q, Luo X, Zhang B, Jiang X, Yi B, and Wu M. Predictive factors for prognosis of hilar cholangiocarcinoma: Postresection radiotherapy improves survival. *Eur J Surg Oncol* 2007; **33**: 202–7.

29. Kayahara M, Nagakawa T, Ohta T, Kitagawa H, Tajima H, and Miwa K. Role of nodal involvement and the periductal soft-tissue margin in middle and distal bile duct cancer. *Ann Surg* 1999; **229**: 76–83.

30. Todoroki T, Kawamoto T, Koike N, Fukao K, Shoda J, and Takahashi H. Treatment strategy for patients with middle and lower third bile duct cancer. *Br J Surg* 2001; **88**: 364–70.

31. Sakamoto Y, Kosuge T, Shimada K, *et al*. Prognostic factors of surgical resection in middle and distal bile duct cancer: An analysis of 55 patients concerning the significance of ductal and radial margins. *Surgery* 2005; **137**: 396–402.

32. Karanicolas PJ, Davies E, Kunz R, *et al*. The pylorus: Take it or leave it? Systematic review and meta-analysis of pylorus-preserving versus standard Whipple pancreaticoduodenectomy for pancreatic or periampullary cancer. *Ann Surg Oncol* 2007; **14**: 1825–34.

33. Cheng Q, Luo X, Zhang B, Jiang X, Yi B, and Wu M. Distal bile duct carcinoma: Prognostic factors after curative surgery. A series of 112 cases. *Ann Surg Oncol* 2006; **14**: 1212–9.

34. Fong Y, Blumgart LH, Lin E, Fortner JG, and Brennan MF. Outcome of treatment for distal bile duct cancer. *Br J Surg* 1996; **83**: 1712–15.

35. Konstadoulakis MM, Roayaie S, Gomatos IP, *et al*. Fifteen-year, single-center experience with the surgical management of intrahepatic cholangiocarcinoma: Operative results and long-term outcome. *Surgery* 2008; **143**: 366–74.

36. Paik KY, Jung JC, Heo JS, Choi SH, Choi DW, and Kim YI. What prognostic factors are important for resected intrahepatic cholangiocarcinoma? *J Gastroenterol Hepatol* 2008; **23**: 766–70.

37. Endo I, Gonen M, Yopp AC, *et al*. Intrahepatic cholangiocarcinoma: Rising frequency, improved survival, and determinants of outcome after resection. *Ann Surg* 2008; **248**: 84–96.

38. Weber SM, Jarnagin WR, Klimstra D, DeMatteo RP, Fong Y, and Blumgart LH. Intrahepatic cholangiocarcinoma: Resectability, recurrence pattern, and outcomes. *J Am Coll Surg* 2001; **193**: 384–91.

39. Pinson CW and Moore DE. Liver transplantation is not indicated for cholangiocarcinoma. *HPB* 2003; **5**: 203–5.

40. Callery M. Transplantation for cholangiocarcinoma: Advance or supply-demand dilemma? *Gastroenterology* 2006; **130**: 2242–4.

41. Brandsaeter B, Isoniemi H, Broome U, *et al*. Liver transplantation for primary sclerosing cholangitis; predictors and consequences of hepatobiliary malignancy. *J Hepatol* 2004; **40**: 815–22.

42. Wu Y, Johlin FC, Rayhill SC, *et al*. Long-term, tumor-free survival after radiotherapy combining hepatectomy-Whipple en bloc and orthotopic liver transplantation for early-stage hilar cholangiocarcinoma. *Liver Transpl* 2008; **14**: 279–86.

43. Ghali P, Marotta PJ, Yoshida EM, *et al*. Liver transplantation for incidental cholangiocarcinoma: Analysis of the Canadian experience. *Liver Transpl* 2005; **11**: 1412–16.

44. Meyer CG, Penn I, and James L. Liver transplantation for cholangiocarcinoma: Results in 207 patients. *Transplantation* 2000; **69**: 1633–7.

45. Kaiser GM, Sotiropoulos GC, Jauch KW, *et al*. Liver transplantation for hilar cholangiocarcinoma: A German survey. *Transplant Proc* 2008; **40**: 3191–3.

46. Becker NS, Rodriguez JA, Barshes NR, O'Mahony CA, Goss JA, and Aloia TA. Outcomes analysis for 280 patients with cholangiocarcinoma treated with liver transplantation over an 18-year period. *J Gastrointest Surg* 2008; **12**: 117–22.

47. Robles R, Figueras J, Turrión VS, *et al.* Liver transplantation for hilar cholangiocarcinoma: Spanish experience. *Transplant Proc* 2003; **35**: 1821–2.

48. Iwatsuki S, Todo S, Marsh JW, *et al.* Treatment of hilar cholangiocarcinoma (Klatskin tumors) with hepatic resection or transplantation. *J Am Coll Surg* 1998; **187**: 358–64.

49. Sotiropoulos GC, Kaiser BM, Lang H, *et al.* Liver transplantation as a primary indication for intrahepatic cholangiocarcinoma: A single center experience. *Transplant Proc* 2008; **40**: 3194–5.

50. Pascher A, Jonas S, and Heuhaus P. Intrahepatic cholangiocarcinoma: Indication for transplantation. *J Hepatobiliary Pancreat Surg* 2003; **10**: 232–7.

51. Robles R, Figueras J, Turrión VS, *et al.* Liver transplantation for peripheral cholangiocarcinoma: Spanish experience. *Transplant Proc* 2003; **35**: 1823–4.

52. Rosen CB, Heimbach JK, and Gores GJ. Surgery for cholangiocarcinoma: The role of liver transplantation. *HPB* 2008; **10**: 186–9.

53. Gores GJ, Nagorney DM, and Rosen CB. Cholangiocarcinoma: Is transplantation an option? For whom? *J Hepatol* 2007; **47**: 455–9.

54. Heimbach JK, Gores GJ, Haddock MG, *et al.* Predictors of disease recurrence following neoadjuvant chemoradiotherapy and liver transplantation for unresectable perihilar cholangiocarcinoma. *Transplantation* 2006; **82**: 1703–7.

55. Neuhaus P, Jonas S, Settmacher U, *et al.* Surgical management of proximal bile duct cancer: Extended right lobe resection increases resectability and radicality. *Langenbecks Arch Surg* 203; **388**: 194–200.

11.2 Non-surgical treatment

a. Radiotherapy

Orit Gutfeld and Charlie Pan

This chapter outlines the available data on the role and use of radiotherapy (RT) in the treatment of biliary malignancies. Adjuvant, definitive, and palliative treatment are discussed for each different site along the biliary tract. The concepts, considerations, and techniques for upper abdominal RT are discussed in detail in Chapter 7.2a.

Postoperative radiotherapy

Surgery is the only potentially curative treatment for patients with biliary carcinoma. However, even with complete resection, the recurrence rate is high and long-term survival is poor. Local recurrence is a common pattern of failure and is associated with significant morbidity and mortality related to hepatobiliary complications. Adjuvant RT can potentially improve local control and survival, but data on its role in this setting are limited. Most of the data are derived from retrospective, single-institution experiences with possible selection bias favoring adjuvant treatments in well-performing patients or in patients with poor prognostic factors. Interpretation of these studies is further complicated by heterogeneity of disease stage, type of resection, and a variety of RT techniques and doses.

Intrahepatic cholangiocarcinoma

Most patients with intrahepatic cholangiocarcinoma (IHC) are not candidates for resection at presentation, mostly because of advanced disease within the liver. After resection, median and 5-year survival are 19 to 37.5 months and 13.6–40%, respectively [1,2,3,4,5,6]. The majority of recurrences involve the liver, either alone

Primary Carcinomas of the Liver, ed. Hero K. Hussain and Isaac R. Francis. Published by Cambridge University Press. © Cambridge University Press 2010.

or in combination with distant sites [1,2,3,4,5,6]. Survival is directly related to the ability to obtain negative surgical margins and the absence of regional lymph-node involvement. There are almost no data on the role of adjuvant RT after resection of IHC. However, in a retrospective series of 30 patients who underwent curative resection of IHC, the use of adjuvant chemoradiation in 9 patients had no impact on survival [3].

A retrospective analysis of 3839 patients with IHC collected from the Surveillance, Epidemiology and End Results (SEER) database suggests that adjuvant RT may prolong survival. Median survival for patients treated with surgery and RT was 11 months, significantly longer than 6 months for patients treated with surgery alone [7]. However, it is possible that patients with an earlier stage of disease and better performance status were selected for adjuvant RT, and therefore the survival benefit may not be a true effect of RT.

Extrahepatic cholangiocarcinoma

Perihilar cholangiocarcinoma

Compared to other locations along the biliary tract, perihilar tumors are associated with a higher proportion of positive margins after resection [8]. In recent years, more aggressive surgeries, including en block partial hepatectomy, have improved the rate of negative resection margins and may have yielded improved survival rates [8,9]. However, even with complete resection and negative margins, 5-year survival rates are 30–52% and local recurrence is high. In a detailed analysis of patterns of failure, isolated local recurrence as the first site of failure was found in as many as 59% of patients [10].

Several retrospective studies have suggested a survival benefit with adjuvant RT after resection of perihilar cholangiocarcinoma. One of the largest studies, by Gerhards *et al.* [11], retrospectively compared the outcomes of 20 patients who received no adjuvant therapy, 41 patients who received external beam radiation therapy (EBRT) and brachytherapy, and 30 patients who received EBRT alone. Median survival was significantly longer in patients who received adjuvant RT: 24 months compared to 8.3 months in the surgery-alone group. Brachytherapy did not contribute to survival and was associated with a higher complication rate. The rate of negative surgical margins in this series was low (14%). Another study from the European Organisation for Research and Treatment of Cancer (EORTC) compared 38 patients who received adjuvant RT after resection of perihilar tumors to 17 patients who were treated with surgery alone. Median survival in the irradiated group was 19 months, significantly longer than 8 months in the surgery-alone group. As in the former series, the majority of patients had positive surgical margins [12].

In contrast, in a prospective, non-randomized analysis of 50 patients who underwent either curative or palliative surgeries for perihilar cholangiocarcinoma, the addition of postoperative RT did not improve survival in either resected or palliated patients. The median survival was 20 months in both groups [13].

Cameron *et al.* [14] analyzed the John Hopkins University experience with 96 patients with perihilar cholangiocarcinoma who were treated surgically with curative resection (41%), non-curative resection (14%), or palliative procedures only (45%). Sixty-three patients (66%) received postoperative EBRT (50–60 Gy); in 31 patients this was followed by brachytherapy (20 Gy). No survival benefit was associated with postoperative RT in the group undergoing curative resection; however, radiation improved survival in patients undergoing palliative surgery. It is possible that the benefit from adjuvant RT is related to margin status with small benefit, or not at all, in patients who had resection with negative margins.

Distal cholangiocarcinoma

Tumors of the distal biliary tract are resectable in up to 90% of cases with a higher probability of achieving negative surgical margins compared to other sites along the biliary tract. Nevertheless, even after negative-margin resection of distal tumors, the 5-year survival is only 27–40%, with median survival of 22 to 25 months [8,15].

In a retrospective study from Johns Hopkins University, 34 patients who underwent pancreaticoduodenectomy for distal common bile-duct tumors received adjuvant RT with concomitant and maintenance 5-fluoruracil (5-FU)–based chemotherapy. The clinical target volume included the tumor bed, the surgical field, the primary lymph-node drainage stations, and paraaortic lymph nodes. Median radiation dose was 50.4 Gy (range 40–54 Gy) in 1.8–2.5 Gy per fraction. Actuarial 5-year local control was 70%. The site of first disease recurrence was local only in 17%, distant in 75%, and both local and distant in 8%. Median overall survival was 37 months with a 5-year survival of 35%, which was better than historical controls of surgery alone. On multivariate analysis, only nodal status significantly predicted survival [16].

Gallbladder carcinoma

The available data on adjuvant RT after resection of gallbladder cancer are limited to small, retrospective, single-institution studies with great heterogeneity in patient selection, treatment techniques, and radiation dose. Although a few studies suggest a survival benefit for postoperative RT, with or without chemotherapy [17,18,19,20,21,22,23], other studies do not confirm such benefit [24,25]. The potential benefit of adjuvant RT is further challenged by detailed analysis of patterns of failure, in which only 15% of patients were found to have isolated locoregional disease as the first site of recurrence [26]. The high rate of negative margin resection (90%) in this analysis may partly explain the much lower rate of local failure compared to other reports and subsequent lack of benefit from adjuvant RT.

In a survival prediction model based upon data from 4180 patients with resected gallbladder cancer who were reported to the SEER database between 1988 and 2003, adjuvant RT was found to provide survival benefit in node-positive or greater than or equal to T2 disease. Median survival for the 760 patients who received RT after resection was 15 months, compared with 8 months for patients who were treated with surgery alone. The model was used to construct a nomogram that can estimate the predicted net survival gain attributable to adjuvant RT, given individual clinical and pathological parameters [27]. However, important parameters such as performance status and surgical margin status were not considered, and the model was not validated prospectively.

Adjuvant radiotherapy: Conclusions

In the absence of high-level evidence, the role of adjuvant RT after resection of biliary tumors remains controversial. Nevertheless, a SEER database analysis of cholangiocarcinoma patients who underwent surgery from 1973 through 2002 has shown an increase in the use of RT in these patients in recent years. Between 1993 and 2002, patients with each stage of disease were more likely to receive RT compared to earlier decades. Yet, in multivariable analysis RT did not show a statistically significant effect on survival [28].

DeOliveira *et al.* [8] analyzed the outcome of 564 cholangiocarcinoma patients who underwent surgery at Johns Hopkins University during a 31-year period (1973–2004). Nearly half (47%) of these patients received RT, with no difference among the three anatomical sites (intrahepatic, perihilar, extrahepatic). Twenty-nine percent of the patients received chemotherapy. There was no statistically significant difference in survival rates between those who received and those who did not receive RT and/or chemotherapy, either in the entire series or in any of the three anatomical sites. RT and/or chemotherapy did not significantly change survival in subgroups of patients who had R0 (negative margin) or R1 and/or R2 resections (microscopic and/or macroscopic residual tumor).

The lack of prospective trials addressing the contribution of adjuvant RT to outcomes in resected biliary cancers makes it difficult to draw definitive conclusions as to benefit. Although there is no standard regimen, the current National Comprehensive Cancer Network (NCCN) guidelines recommend consideration of adjuvant fluoropyrimidine chemoradiation in cases of IHC with positive surgical margins, in EHCC, especially if margins are positive or if regional lymph nodes are involved, and in any gallbladder carcinoma greater than or equal to T2 or N1, regardless of margin status [29].

Neoadjuvant therapy

Neoadjuvant chemoradiation may potentially downstage unresectable tumors and render them resectable. The potential benefit of this approach for selected patients was demonstrated in a retrospective series from the M.D. Anderson Cancer Center, in which nine patients with EHCC (five perihilar, four distal) underwent chemoradiation prior to resection. Treatment consisted of EBRT (30–50.4 Gy in 1.8–3 Gy per fraction) with concomitant administration of continuous 5-FU. Three of the patients had a pathologic complete response, whereas the remainder showed different degrees of response. All 9 patients had negative surgical margins, compared to a negative margin rate of 54% in the 31 patients who underwent curative resections up-front. However, there was no survival difference among the patients who received neoadjuvant treatment, those who received postoperative chemoradiation, and those who did not receive RT at all [30].

Neoadjuvant treatment and transplantation

Early experience with liver transplantation for cholangiocarcinoma was uniformly disappointing, with high recurrence rates and 5-year survival of only ~20% at best.

However, a 5-year survival rate of 82% was reported by Rea *et al.* [31] in a series of 38 patients with hilar cholangiocarcinoma who underwent liver transplantation after neoadjuvant chemoradiation. The treatment consisted of EBRT (45 Gy in 30 fractions), concomitant chemotherapy (5-FU), and intraluminal brachytherapy (ILBT; 20–30 Gy) followed by formal staging procedure to rule out extrahepatic disease before proceeding to transplantation [31]. In a smaller series from Nebraska Medical Center using a similar strategy, long-term, tumor-free survival was achieved in 45% of the transplanted patients [32]. Such an approach may be considered for highly selected patients and as part of a clinical trial at specialized centers.

Locally advanced disease

The majority of patients with biliary tumors present with advanced disease that is not amenable to surgery. Several retrospective studies suggest that RT, with or without chemotherapy, may palliate symptoms and prolong survival of patients with non-metastatic, locally advanced disease [33,34,35,36,37,38].

Radiotherapy considerations

In Phase I and II trials from the University of Michigan, 128 patients with unresectable hepatic malignancies were treated with conformal RT (median dose 60.75 Gy in twice-daily, 1.5-Gy fractions) with concurrent hepatic arterial floxuridine. The median survival of the 46 patients with IHC in this study was 13.3 months. On multivariable analysis, the total radiation dose was found to be the only significant predictor of survival. Patients who received doses greater than or equal to 75 Gy had significantly higher overall survival than those receiving lower doses [39].

Delivery of higher radiation doses to the biliary tract is limited by the radiation tolerance of adjacent organs – mainly the liver, stomach, duodenum, and kidneys. ILBT uses a radioactive source (I-192) that is inserted into the tumor-bearing area through a biliary drainage catheter. This technique allows the focal delivery of high radiation doses to the tumor but spares adjacent normal tissues, due to a steep dose gradient over a short distance from the radioactive source. Brachytherapy is frequently used for EHCC to supplement EBRT. Typical doses delivered with brachytherapy range from 15 to 30 Gy prescribed to 0.5 to 1.0 cm from the source. Retrospective studies suggest improved survival with the combined approach. A summary of studies using EBRT alone or in combination with brachytherapy and/or chemotherapy is given in Table 11.2a.1. It should be noted that ILBT may also increase the risk of long-term complications.

Table 11.2a.1 Selected results of RT for unresectable biliary cancer

No. of patients/Site of disease	Treatment	Median survival (months)	Overall survival	Local control	Long-term toxicity (No. of patients)
Grove et al. [33] 19/hilar 9/hilar	19 EBRT (12.6–64 Gy) 9 palliative surgery alone	12.2 2.2	Not reported	Not reported	Not reported
Crane et al. [34] 52/EHCC	EBRT (30–85 Gy/1.8–3 Gy per fraction) Concomitant 5-FU in 38 pts (73%) 4 pts received ILBT or intraoperative boost (20 Gy)	10	13% at 2 years	41% at 1 year	Duodenal ulcer (1) Cholangitis (3)
Brunner et al. [35] 64/EHCC (5 pts with gallbladder carcinoma)	25 EBRT (45–50.4 Gy in 1.8 Gy/fraction) + ILBT (10 Gy) Concomitant 5-FU and mitomycin (10 pts), or concomitant gemcitabine and cisplatin (14 pts) 39 palliative stenting	16.5 9.3	Not reported	Not reported	Not reported
Foo et al. [36] 24/EHCC	EBRT (median dose 50.4 Gy in 1.8-Gy fractions) ILBT (median dose 20 Gy at 1 cm) Concomitant 5-FU in 9 pts	12.8	14.4% at 5 years	67%	Cholangitis (12) Biliary stricture (1) Duodenal ulcers with upper GI bleeding (10) Gastric/duodenal obstruction (3)
Morganti at al. [37] 20/EHCC	EBRT (39.6–50.4 Gy) ILBT (12 pts; 30–50 Gy at 1 cm) Concomitant 5-FU (19 pts)	21.2	14.7% at 5 years	Not reported	GI ulcers (2)
Takamura et al. [38] 93/EHCC	EBRT (50 Gy in 2-Gy fractions) ILBT (27–50 Gy at 0.5 cm)	11.9	4% at 5 years	56%	GI bleeding (19) Biliary complications (31)

GI, gastrointestinal tract.

A different technique to increase the biologic equivalent dose to the target is stereotactic body radiation therapy (SBRT), in which highly precise targeting and dose delivery allow potent ablative doses to be delivered to the target with either a single fraction or a small number of fractions. (For a more detailed description of this technique, please refer to Chapter 7.2a.) Ten patients with IHC were treated in a Phase I study of SBRT for primary liver malignancies. The median prescription dose was 36.0 Gy (24–54 Gy) given in six fractions. The median and 1-year survival for IHC were 15 months and 58%. The 1-year in-field local control rate was 65% with hepatic out-of-field recurrence being the most frequent site of first failure [40].

Summary and future directions

Multiple retrospective trials suggest a benefit from RT administration in biliary malignancies, both in the adjuvant setting and as a definitive or palliative treatment in selected patients with advanced disease. Randomized controlled trials are needed to better define the role of RT in the management of biliary cancer and to better select the patients who are most likely to benefit from it. The optimal RT technique and fractionation and combinations with other modalities should also be investigated in a prospective randomized manner. Given the rarity of this disease, such trials require multiinstitutional and probably international collaboration.

Although the results with newer radiation techniques and combined therapies are promising, the high rate of locoregional failures and the poor overall survival after treatment underscore the need for novel therapeutic strategies for biliary malignancies.

Possible approaches are further escalation of the radiation dose by using high-precision radiation techniques such as intensity-modulated radiation therapy (IMRT), SBRT, and charged-particle RT (see Chapter 7.2a). Combining RT with more potent radiosensitizers may also improve the outcome. Targeted agents such as inhibitors of the epidermal growth factor receptor (EGFR) or the vascular endothelial growth factor (VEGF) pathways may be good candidates for such a combined approach.

Most patients with biliary cancer present with advanced disease. In patients who have limited local disease, therapies such as surgery and RT provide cure in only a minority of patients. It is obvious that an effective systemic therapy is needed. Our hope is that better understanding of the etiology and molecular pathogenesis of biliary cancer will lead to the development of such treatment.

REFERENCES

1. Endo I, Gonen M, Yopp AC, *et al.* Intrahepatic cholangiocarcinoma: Rising frequency, improved survival, and determinants of outcome after resection. *Ann Surg* 2008; **248**(1): 84–96.

2. Isa T, Kusano T, Shimoji H, Takeshima Y, Muto Y, and Furukawa M. Predictive factors for long-term survival in patients with intrahepatic cholangiocarcinoma. *Am J Surg* 2001; **181**(6): 507–11.

3. Valverde A, Bonhomme N, Ferges O, *et al.* Resection of intrahepatic cholangiocarcinoma: A western experience. *J Hepatobiliary Pancreat Surg* 1999; **6**: 122–7.

4. Madariaga JR, Iwatsuki S, Todo S, Lee RG, Irish W, and Starzl TE. Liver resection for hilar and peripheral cholangiocarcinomas: A study of 62 cases. *Ann Surg* 1998; **227**(1): 70–9.

5. Jan YY, Yeh CN, Yeh TS, Hwang TL, and Chen MF. Clinicopathological factors predicting long-term overall survival after hepatectomy for peripheral cholangiocarcinoma. *World J Surg* 2005; **29**(7): 894–8.

6. Weber SM, Jarnagin WR, Klimstra D, DeMatteo RP, Fong Y, and Blumgart LH. Intrahepatic cholangiocarcinoma: Resectability, recurrence pattern, and outcomes. *J Am Coll Surg* 2001; **193**(4): 384–91.

7. Shinohara ET, Mitra N, Guo M, and Metz JM. Radiation therapy is associated with improved survival in the adjuvant and definitive treatment of intrahepatic cholangiocarcinoma. *Int J Radiat Oncol Biol Phys* 2008; **72**(5): 1495–501.

8. DeOliveira ML, Cunningham SC, Cameron JL, *et al.* Cholangiocarcinoma: Thirty-one-year experience with 564 patients at a single institution. *Ann Surg* 2007; **245**(5): 755–62.

9. Kosuge T, Yamamoto J, Shimada K, Yamasaki S, and Makuuchi M. Improved surgical results for hilar cholangiocarcinoma with procedures including major hepatic resection. *Ann Surg* 1999; **230**(5): 663–71.

10. Jarnagin WR, Fong Y, DeMatteo RP, *et al.* Staging, resectability, and outcome in 225 patients with hilar cholangiocarcinoma. *Ann Surg* 2001; **234**(4): 507–17.

11. Gerhards MF, van Gulik TM, Gonzáles Gonzáles D, Rauws EA, and Gouma DJ. Results of postoperative radiotherapy for resectable hilar cholangiocarcinoma. *World J Surg* 2003; **27**(2): 173–9.

12. Gonzáles Gonzáles D, Gerard J, Maners AW, *et al.* Results of radiation therapy in carcinoma of the proximal bile duct (Klatskin tumor). *Semin Liver Dis* 1990; **10**(2): 131–41.

13. Pitt HA, Nakeeb A, Abrams RA, *et al.* Perihilar cholangiocarcinoma: Postoperative radiotherapy does not improve survival. *Ann Surg* 1995; **221**(6): 788–97.

14. Cameron JL, Pitt HA, Zinner MJ, Kaufman SL, and Coleman J. Management of proximal cholangiocarcinomas by surgical resection and radiotherapy. *Am J Surg* 1990; **159**(1): 91–7.

15. Nakeeb A and Pitt HA. Radiation therapy, chemotherapy and chemoradiation in hilar cholangiocarcinoma. *HPB* (Oxford) 2005; **7**(4): 278–82.

16. Hughes MA, Frassica DA, Yeo CJ, *et al.* Adjuvant concurrent chemoradiation for adenocarcinoma of the distal common bile duct. *Int J Radiat Oncol Biol Phys* 2007; **68**(1): 178–82.

17. Kresl JJ, Schild SE, Henning GT, *et al.* Adjuvant external beam radiation therapy with concurrent chemotherapy in the management of gallbladder carcinoma. *Int J Radiat Oncol Biol Phys* 2002; **52**(1): 167–75.

18. Mahe M, Stampfli C, Romestaing P, and Salerno N. Primary carcinoma of the gall-bladder: Potential for external radiation therapy. *Radiother Oncol* 1994; **33**: 204.

19. Nakeeb A, Tran KQ, Black MJ, *et al.* Improved survival in resected biliary malignancies. *Surgery* 2002; **132**: 555.

20. Ben-David MA, Griffith KA, Abu-Isa E, *et al.* External-beam radiotherapy for localized extrahepatic cholangiocarcinoma. *Int J Radiat Oncol Biol Phys* 2006; **66**(3): 772–9.

21. Houry S, Barrier A, and Huguier M. Irradiation therapy for gallbladder carcinoma: Recent advances. *J Hepatobiliary Pancreat Surg* 2001; **8**(6): 518–24.

22. Todoroki T, Kawamoto T, Otsuka M, *et al.* Benefits of combining radiotherapy with aggressive resection for Stage IV gallbladder cancer. *Hepato-Gastroenterology* 1999; **46**(27): 1585–91.

23. Czito BG, Hurwitz HI, Clough RW, *et al.* Adjuvant external-beam radiotherapy with concurrent chemotherapy after resection of primary gallbladder carcinoma: A 23-year experience. *Int J Radiat Oncol Biol Phys* 2005; **62**(4): 1030–4.

24. Itoh H, Nishijima K, Kurosaka Y, *et al.* Magnitude of combination therapy of radical resection and external beam radiotherapy for patients with carcinomas of the extrahepatic bile duct and gallbladder. *Dig Dis Sci* 2005; **50**(12): 2231–42.

25. Chao TC and Greager JA. Primary carcinoma of the gallbladder. *J Surg Oncol* 1991; **46**(4): 215–21.

26. Jarnagin WR, Ruo L, Little SA, *et al.* Patterns of initial disease recurrence after resection of gallbladder carcinoma and hilar cholangiocarcinoma: Implications for adjuvant therapeutic strategies. *Cancer* 2003; **98**(8): 1689–700.

27. Wang SJ, Fuller CD, Kim JS, Sittig DF, Thomas CR, and Ravdin PM. Prediction model for estimating the survival benefit of adjuvant radiotherapy for gallbladder cancer. *J Clin Oncol* 2008; **26**(13): 2112–17.

28. Nathan H, Pawlik TM, Wolfgang CL, Choti MA, Cameron JL, and Schulick RD. Trends in survival after surgery for cholangiocarcinoma: A 30-year population-based SEER database analysis. *J Gastrointest Surg* 2007; **11**(11): 1488–97.

29. National Cancer Comprehensive Network (NCCN). NCCN clinical practice guidelines in oncology, hepatobiliary cancers V.2.2009. Available from: http://www.*nccn.org/professionals/physician_gls/PDF/hepatobiliary.pdf*. Accessed August 5, 2009.

30. McMasters KM, Tuttle TM, Leach SD, *et al.* Neoadjuvant chemoradiation for extrahepatic cholangiocarcinoma. *Am J Surg* 1997; **174**(6): 605–8; discussion 608–9.

31. Rea DJ, Heimbach JK, Rosen CB, *et al.* Liver transplantation with neoadjuvant chemoradiation is more effective than resection for hilar cholangiocarcinoma. *Ann Surg* 2005; **242**(3): 451–8; discussion 458–61.

32. Sudan D, DeRoover A, Chinnakotla S, *et al*. Radiochemotherapy and transplantation allow long-term survival for nonresectable hilar cholangiocarcinoma. *Am J Transplant* 2002; **2**(8): 774–9.

33. Grove MK, Hermann RE, Vogt DP, and Broughan TA. Role of radiation after operative palliation in cancer of the proximal bile ducts. *Am J Surg* 1991; **161**(4): 454–8.

34. Crane CH, Macdonald KO, Vauthey JN, *et al*. Limitations of conventional doses of chemoradiation for unresectable biliary cancer. *Int J Radiat Oncol Biol Phys* 2002; **53**(4): 969–74.

35. Brunner TB, Schwab D, Meyer T, and Sauer R. Chemoradiation may prolong survival of patients with non-bulky unresectable extrahepatic biliary carcinoma. A retrospective analysis. *Strahlenther Onkol* 2004; **180**(12): 751–7.

36. Foo ML, Gunderson LL, Bender CE, and Buskirk SJ. External radiation therapy and transcatheter iridium in the treatment of extrahepatic bile duct carcinoma. *Int J Radiat Oncol Biol Phys* 1997; **39**(4): 929–35.

37. Morganti AG, Trodella L, Valentini V, *et al*. Combined modality treatment in unresectable extrahepatic biliary carcinoma. *Int J Radiat Oncol Biol Phys* 2000; **46**(4): 913–19.

38. Takamura A, Saito H, Kamada T, *et al*. Intraluminal low-dose-rate Ir-192 brachytherapy combined with external beam radiotherapy and biliary stenting For unresectable extrahepatic bile duct carcinoma. *Int J Radiat Oncol Biol Phys* 2003; **57**(5): 1357–65.

39. Ben-Josef E, Normolle D, Ensminger WD, *et al*. Phase II trial of high-dose conformal radiation therapy with concurrent hepatic artery floxuridine for unresectable intrahepatic malignancies. *J Clin Oncol* 2005; **23**(34): 8739–47.

40. Tse RV, Hawkins M, Lockwood G, *et al*. Phase I study of individualized stereotactic body radiotherapy for hepatocellular carcinoma and intrahepatic cholangiocarcinoma. *J Clin Oncol* 2008; **26**(4): 657–64.

b. Systemic therapy

Gazala N. Khan and Mark M. Zalupski

Introduction

Cholangiocarcinoma is an uncommon malignancy, arising from the intra- or extra-hepatic biliary system or gallbladder. In general, this cancer is associated with a poor prognosis, with an estimated 5-year survival rate of approximately 10%. Complete surgical resection provides the only potentially curative option. Unfortunately, the majority of cases are locally advanced or metastatic at initial diagnosis and, therefore, beyond effective surgical treatment. Advanced cholangiocarcinoma may be treated with systemic chemotherapy. Prospective clinical trial data in this disease regarding systemic treatment are limited and generally restricted to Phase II experiences. Given the similarities of histologic appearance and clinical behavior of cholangiocarcinoma and pancreatic cancer, treatment used in pancreatic cancer has been employed in cholangiocarcinoma. Increased understanding of the underlying tumor biology of cholangiocarcinoma and the advent of targeted biologic agents toward cancer-specific pathways hold the promise of improved therapy for this uncommon disease.

Chemotherapy for resected cholangiocarcinoma

Following complete surgical resection of cholangiocarcinoma, as many as 60% of patients will develop recurrent disease. In other resected cancers, use of chemotherapy in the postoperative or adjuvant setting has been shown to delay or prevent disease recurrence. However, in cholangiocarcinoma, there is a paucity of data regarding the use of adjuvant chemotherapy. A single randomized, multicenter trial using 5-fluorouracil (5-FU) and mitomycin C demonstrated a 13% difference in 5-year survival rates, favoring treated patients; however, this difference did not reach statistical significance [1]. Thus, the role of adjuvant chemotherapy in

Primary Carcinomas of the Liver, ed. Hero K. Hussain and Isaac R. Francis. Published by Cambridge University Press. © Cambridge University Press 2010.

resected cholangiocarcinoma remains to be defined. The primary use of chemotherapy in cholangiocarcinoma is in the advanced or metastatic setting and is given with palliative intent.

Chemotherapy for advanced cholangiocarcinoma

Chemotherapy in advanced cholangiocarcinoma is used primarily to control disease and alleviate or palliate symptoms. Early reports of chemotherapy in cholangiocarcinoma from the late 1970s through the 1980s were small studies and demonstrated modest and uncertain benefits of chemotherapy [2,3,4,5]. Subsequently, in the mid-1990s, it was suggested that chemotherapy led to an improvement in quality-of-life (QOL) measures and also appeared to improve survival. In one randomized controlled trial it was shown that 36% of patients with cholangiocarcinoma treated with 5-FU–based chemotherapy had stable or improved QOL parameters as compared to only 10% in the supportive care group ($p < 0.01$). In addition, median survival was increased in patients receiving chemotherapy from 2.5 months to 6 months ($p < 0.01$) [6]. This important trial supported treatment of patients with cholangiocarcinoma due to observed palliative and survival benefits. Over the past decade, additional studies have been conducted evaluating the role of other cytotoxic agents in this disease. The results of selected studies are summarized in Table 11.2b.1. The most active single agents appear to be 5-FU and gemcitabine. The remainder of this chapter provides an overview of more recent trials that define chemotherapy use in this disease. In addition, a potential role for targeted therapy is highlighted.

Fluoropyrimidine-based regimens

Studies using 5-FU as a single agent in cholangiocarcinoma have reported benefits analogous to the Glimelius *et al.* [6] study discussed above [4,7]. Given that single-agent 5-FU appeared to be associated with benefit in this disease, combinations of 5-FU with other chemotherapy drugs, primarily platinum analogues, or the biologic agent interferon were performed. A preferred mode of administration of 5-FU is intravenous continuous infusion typically administered over hours to several days. Most of the combination studies in cholangiocarcinoma have employed infusional 5-FU.

Cisplatin has been combined with 5-FU resulting in 24 and 34% partial response rates [8,9] and was well tolerated with minimal toxicity. The addition of epirubicin

Table 11.2b.1 Single agent and combination chemotherapeutic regimens in cholangiocarcinoma, selected studies[a]

Regimen	N	Median survival (months)	Response rate (%)	Progression-free survival (months)	Comments
5-FU/LV/Eto [6]	37	6.5	11.0	3.5	Improved QOL
5-FU/Cis [8]	25	10.0	24.0	NR	
5-FU/Cis/Epi [10]	20	11.0	40.0	10.0	Minimal toxicity
5-FU/Cis/Epi [11]	20	5.0	10.0	2.0	Continuous infusion 5-FU
Gem [22]	32	11.5	22.0	5.6	2200 mg/m^2 q2w
Gem/5-FU [23]	42	9.7	9.5	4.6	Benefit equivalent to Gem alone
Gem/Cis [26]	43	9.0	27.5	5.1	Cis q3w
Gem/Ox [29]	31	11.0	26.0	6.5	Ox dosed q15 days
Gem/Doc [32]	43	11.0	9.0	5.2	Doc 35mg^2 weekly for 3 weeks
Gem/Iri [31]	14	NR	14.0	NR	Preliminary report – ongoing
Gem/Cap [17]	45	14.0	33.0	7.0	47% with gallbladder cancer

[a] LV, leucovorin; Cis, cisplatin; Gem, gemcitabine; Eto, etoposide; Epi, epirubicin; Ox, oxaliplatin; Dox, docetaxel; Iri, irinotecan; Cap, capecitabine; NR, none reported; q2w, every 2 weeks.

to infusional 5-FU and cisplatin (ECF) has also been evaluated in advanced biliary cancer. Reported response rates in patients treated with ECF range from 10 to 40%. Median progression-free survival intervals have ranged from 2 to 10 months. This regimen was well tolerated with minimal toxicity [10,11]. Etoposide has been added to ECF as part of a four-drug regimen and has been tested in biliary cancer; however, this combination appeared to be more toxic compared to ECF alone [12]. Interferon has also been combined with infusional 5-FU and cisplatin. However, this combination appears to have no additional benefit and also demonstrated increased toxicity [13,14]. Currently, the combination of 5-FU and cisplatin, with or without epirubicin, has modest activity in this disease, is well tolerated, and might be considered as first-line therapy in patients with advanced cholangiocarcinoma.

Capecitabine is an orally administered 5-FU prodrug, which after ingestion undergoes a three-step metabolic activation to 5-FU. Pharmacokinetic studies and clinical toxicities of capecitabine mimic those of infusional 5-FU. Capecitabine has been studied in cholangiocarcinoma in combination with epirubicin and cisplatin (ECX). This three-drug combination was well tolerated and appears active with a reported response rate of 40% and a median survival of 8 months [15]. Capecitabine has been studied as a single agent in a small series of 18 patients with cholangiocarcinoma demonstrating a modest response rate of 6% [16]. However, in combination with other cytotoxic chemotherapeutic agents, capecitabine is likely to assume a larger role in systemic treatment of cholangiocarcinoma [17].

Gemcitabine-based regimens

Gemcitabine is a pyrimidine analogue that is phosphorylated intracellularly and inhibits ribonucleotide reductase and subsequently deoxyribonucleic acid (DNA) synthesis. A pivotal study in pancreatic cancer randomized 126 patients with advanced, symptomatic disease to either weekly gemcitabine or bolus 5-FU using clinical benefit as the primary endpoint. The study reported advantages in clinical benefit (24% vs. 5%) and median survival (5.6 vs. 4.4 months) favoring gemcitabine [18]. Appreciating the relationship of pancreatic cancer and cholangiocarcinoma, gemcitabine has been evaluated in cholangiocarcinoma.

At least four studies have reported gemcitabine as a single agent in cholangiocarcinoma, with response rates ranging from 6 to 30% and median survivals of 7.5 to 13.1 months [19,20,21,22]. Toxicity was mild. Additional trials evaluating gemcitabine in combination with other chemotherapy agents have been performed. Gemcitabine and bolus 5-FU (given over 1 hour) appeared to have no significant advantage over single-agent gemcitabine [23]. Whether providing 5-FU by infusion would improve this result is unknown. Capecitabine has been combined with gemcitabine in several studies [17,24,25]. These data suggest improved efficacy with response rates ranging from 29 to 32%, and median survivals of 12.7 to 14.0 months. Based on these experiences, capecitabine is often substituted for 5-FU in combination with gemcitabine.

Gemcitabine in combination with a platinum compound also appears promising. In a number of clinical investigations, gemcitabine with cisplatin or oxaliplatin appears to be well tolerated and demonstrates incremental benefit over gemcitabine alone. In a series of studies using gemcitabine and cisplatin, response rates have ranged from 27 to 34% and median survival from 9 to 11 months [26,27,28]. The combination of gemcitabine and oxaliplatin has produced similar results, with a reported response rate of 26% and an overall survival duration of 11 months in one study [29].

Gemcitabine has been combined with the topoisomerase inhibitor irinotecan with some benefit. The incidence of therapy-related neutropenia with this combination was increased, however, and other combinations are seemingly better tolerated [30,31]. The taxanes, paclitaxel and docetaxel, are not active as single agents but may be useful in combination with gemcitabine as has been reported in pancreatic cancer [32,33,34].

Evolving role of targeted therapy

An emerging area of therapeutic research in oncology is the advent of targeted agents, designed and developed to antagonize cancer-specific pathways that drive the malignant phenotype. These targets are often oncogenes, such as the epidermal growth factor receptor (EGFR), which are overexpressed or overactive in tumors and the inhibition of which may lead to a wide array of therapeutic effects manifest by clinical benefit in vivo.

Erlotinib is a potent, small-molecule, tyrosine kinase inhibitor that inhibits the intracellular catalytic domain of EGFR [35]. EGFR expression has been shown to be increased in cholangiocarcinoma [36]. In one study, 42 patients with cholangio-carcinoma underwent therapy with single-agent erlotinib at an oral dose of 150 mg daily. Three partial responses were noted with seven patients remaining progression-free at 6 months [37]. As has been observed in other malignancies, combinations of EGFR inhibitors with chemotherapy or other biologic agents might be associated with increased benefit and need to be evaluated. Lapatinib, a dual inhibitor of EGFR and human epidermal growth factor receptor 2 (HER2), has been tested in Phase II trials in cholangiocarcinoma. No objective responses were observed, although 5 of 17 patients in one study had evidence of disease stability on serial imaging [38].

Angiogenesis, and the vascular endothelial growth pathway (VEGF) in particular, have been targeted for treatment in advanced cancer. The VEGF pathway has been identified as overexpressed and associated with a poor prognosis in cholangiocarci-noma [39]. Bevacizumab, a monoclonal antibody that binds circulating VEGF and effectively depletes it from circulation impairing angiogenesis, is under investigation in this disease. Oral tyrosine kinase inhibitors, such as sorafenib and sunitinib, which interfere with VEGF signaling in cancer cells and peritumoral endothelial cells, are also under study.

Conclusion

Cholangiocarcinoma is an uncommon disease and, in an advanced stage, is associated with a poor prognosis. Further study of this disease with regard to its underlying biology, as well as continued evaluation of available and emerging systemic therapies, is urgently needed. In advanced cholangiocarcinoma, systemic therapy with either 5-FU– or gemcitabine-based combination therapy is associated with an improvement in QOL and a modest survival benefit. Better understanding of the prognostic and predictive parameters in individual patients may assist in defining optimal systemic treatment.

REFERENCES

1. Takada T, Amano H, Yasuda H, *et al.* Is postoperative adjuvant chemotherapy useful for gallbladder carcinoma? A phase III multicenter prospective randomized controlled trial in patients with resected pancreaticobiliary carcinoma. *Cancer* 2002; **95**(8): 1685–95.

2. Kajanti M and Pyrhonen S. Epirubicin-sequential methotrexate-5-fluorouracil-leucovorin treatment in advanced cancer of the extrahepatic biliary system. A phase II study. *Am J Clin Oncol* 1994; **17**(3): 223–6.

3. Harvey JH, Smith FP, and Schein PS. 5-Fluorouracil, mitomycin, and doxorubicin (FAM) in carcinoma of the biliary tract. *J Clin Oncol* 1984; **2**(11): 1245–8.

4. Falkson G, MacIntyre JM, and Moertel CG. Eastern Cooperative Oncology Group experience with chemotherapy for inoperable gallbladder and bile duct cancer. *Cancer* 1984; **54**(6): 965–9.

5. Takada T, Kato H, Matsushiro T, Nimura Y, Nagakawa T, and Nakayama T. Comparison of 5-fluorouracil, doxorubicin and mitomycin C with 5-fluorouracil alone in the treatment of pancreatic-biliary carcinomas. *Oncology* 1994; **51**(5): 396–400.

6. Glimelius B, Hoffman K, Sjoden PO, *et al.* Chemotherapy improves survival and quality of life in advanced pancreatic and biliary cancer. *Ann Oncol* 1996; **7**(6): 593–600.

7. Davis HL, Jr., Ramirez G, and Ansfield FJ. Adenocarcinomas of stomach, pancreas, liver, and biliary tracts. Survival of 328 patients treated with fluoropyrimidine therapy. *Cancer* 1974; **33**(1): 193–7.

8. Ducreux M, Rougier P, Fandi A, *et al.* Effective treatment of advanced biliary tract carcinoma using 5-fluorouracil continuous infusion with cisplatin. *Ann Oncol* 1998; **9**(6): 653–6.

9. Taieb J, Mitry E, Boige V, *et al.* Optimization of 5-fluorouracil (5-FU)/cisplatin combination chemotherapy with a new schedule of leucovorin, 5-FU and cisplatin (LV5FU2-P regimen) in patients with biliary tract carcinoma. *Ann Oncol* 2002; **13**(8): 1192–6.

10. Ellis PA, Norman A, Hill A, *et al.* Epirubicin, cisplatin and infusional 5-fluorouracil (5-FU) (ECF) in hepatobiliary tumours. *Eur J Cancer* 1995; **31A**(10): 1594–8.

11. Lee MA, Woo IS, Kang JH, Hong YS, and Lee KS. Epirubicin, cisplatin, and protracted infusion of 5-FU (ECF) in advanced intrahepatic cholangiocarcinoma. *J Cancer Res Clin Oncol* 2004; **130**(6): 346–50.

12. Rao S, Cunningham D, Hawkins RE, *et al.* Phase III study of 5FU, etoposide and leucovorin (FELV) compared to epirubicin, cisplatin and 5FU (ECF) in previously untreated patients with advanced biliary cancer. *Br J Cancer* 2005; **92**(9): 1650–4.

13. Patt YZ, Hassan MM, Lozano RD, *et al.* Phase II trial of cisplatin, interferon alpha-2b, doxorubicin, and 5-fluorouracil for biliary tract cancer. *Clin Cancer Res* 2001; **7**(11): 3375–80.

14. Patt YZ, Jones DV, Jr., Hoque A, *et al.* Phase II trial of intravenous fluorouracil and subcutaneous interferon alfa-2b for biliary tract cancer. *J Clin Oncol* 1996; **14**(8): 2311–15.

15. Park SH, Park YH, Lee JN, *et al.* Phase II study of epirubicin, cisplatin, and capecitabine for advanced biliary tract adenocarcinoma. *Cancer* 2006; **106**(2): 361–5.

16. Patt YZ, Hassan MM, Aguayo A, *et al.* Oral capecitabine for the treatment of hepatocellular carcinoma, cholangiocarcinoma, and gallbladder carcinoma. *Cancer* 2004; **101**(3): 578–86.

17. Knox JJ, Hedley D, Oza A, *et al.* Combining gemcitabine and capecitabine in patients with advanced biliary cancer: A phase II trial. *J Clin Oncol* 2005; **23**(10): 2332–8.

18. Burris H and Storniolo AM. Assessing clinical benefit in the treatment of pancreas cancer: Gemcitabine compared to 5-fluorouracil. *Eur J Cancer* 1997; **33**(Suppl 1): S18–22.

19. Tsavaris N, Kosmas C, Gouveris P, *et al.* Weekly gemcitabine for the treatment of biliary tract and gallbladder cancer. *Invest New Drugs* 2004; **22**(2): 193–8.

20. Park JS, Oh SY, Kim SH, *et al.* Single-agent gemcitabine in the treatment of advanced biliary tract cancers: A phase II study. *Jpn J Clin Oncol* 2005; **35**(2): 68–73.

21. von Delius S, Lersch C, Schulte-Frohlinde E, Mayr M, Schmid RM, and Eckel F. Phase II trial of weekly 24-hour infusion of gemcitabine in patients with advanced gallbladder and biliary tract carcinoma. *BMC Cancer* 2005; **5**(1): 61.

22. Penz M, Kornek GV, Raderer M, *et al.* Phase II trial of two-weekly gemcitabine in patients with advanced biliary tract cancer. *Ann Oncol* 2001; **12**(2): 183–6.

23. Alberts SR, Al-Khatib H, Mahoney MR, *et al.* Gemcitabine, 5-fluorouracil, and leucovorin in advanced biliary tract and gallbladder carcinoma: A North Central Cancer Treatment Group phase II trial. *Cancer* 2005; **103**(1): 111–18.

24. Riechelmann RP, Townsley CA, Chin SN, Pond GR, and Knox JJ. Expanded phase II trial of gemcitabine and capecitabine for advanced biliary cancer. *Cancer* 2007; **110**(6): 1307–12.

25. Cho JY, Paik YH, Chang YS, *et al.* Capecitabine combined with gemcitabine (CapGem) as first-line treatment in patients with advanced/metastatic biliary tract carcinoma. *Cancer* 2005; **104**(12): 2753–8.

26. Thongprasert S, Napapan S, Charoentum C, and Moonprakan S. Phase II study of gemcitabine and cisplatin as first-line chemotherapy in inoperable biliary tract carcinoma. *Ann Oncol* 2005; **16**(2): 279–81.

27. Park BK, Kim YJ, Park JY, *et al.* Phase II study of gemcitabine and cisplatin in advanced biliary tract cancer. *J Gastroenterol Hepatol* 2006; **21**(6): 999–1003.

28. Kim ST, Park JO, Lee J, *et al.* A Phase II study of gemcitabine and cisplatin in advanced biliary tract cancer. *Cancer* 2006; **106**(6): 1339–46.

29. Harder J, Riecken B, Kummer O, *et al.* Outpatient chemotherapy with gemcitabine and oxaliplatin in patients with biliary tract cancer. *Br J Cancer* 2006; **95**(7): 848–52.

30. Sanz-Altamira PM, O'Reilly E, Stuart KE, *et al.* A phase II trial of irinotecan (CPT-11) for unresectable biliary tree carcinoma. *Ann Oncol* 2001; **12**(4): 501–4.

31. Bhargava P, Jani CR, Savarese DM, O'Donnell JL, Stuart KE, and Rocha Lima CM. Gemcitabine and irinotecan in locally advanced or metastatic biliary cancer: Preliminary report. *Oncology* (Williston Park) 2003; **17**(9 Suppl 8): 23–6.

32. Kuhn R, Hribaschek A, Eichelmann K, Rudolph S, Fahlke J, and Ridwelski K. Outpatient therapy with gemcitabine and docetaxel for gallbladder, biliary, and cholangio-carcinomas. *Invest New Drugs* 2002; **20**(3): 351–6.

33. Papakostas P, Kouroussis C, Androulakis N, *et al.* First-line chemotherapy with docetaxel for unresectable or metastatic carcinoma of the biliary tract. A multicentre phase II study. *Eur J Cancer* 2001; **37**(15): 1833–8.

34. Jones DV, Jr., Lozano R, Hoque A, Markowitz A, and Patt YZ. Phase II study of paclitaxel therapy for unresectable biliary tree carcinomas. *J Clin Oncol* 1996; **14**(8): 2306–10.

35. Woodburn JR. The epidermal growth factor receptor and its inhibition in cancer therapy. *Pharmacol Ther* 1999; **82**(2–3): 241–50.

36. Lee CS and Pirdas A. Epidermal growth factor receptor immunoreactivity in gallbladder and extrahepatic biliary tract tumours. *Pathol Res Pract* 1995; **191**(11): 1087–91.

37. Philip PA, Mahoney MR, Allmer C, *et al.* Phase II study of erlotinib in patients with advanced biliary cancer. *J Clin Oncol* 2006; **24**(19): 3069–74.

38. Hezel AF and Zhu AX. Systemic therapy for biliary tract cancers. *Oncologist* 2008; **13**(4): 415–23.

39. Hida Y, Morita T, Fujita M, *et al.* Vascular endothelial growth factor expression is an independent negative predictor in extrahepatic biliary tract carcinomas. *Anticancer Res* 1999; **19**(3B): 2257–60.

12

Uncommon hepatic tumors

Peter S. Liu and Hero K. Hussain

Although hepatocellular carcinoma (HCC) and cholangiocarcinoma comprise the majority of malignant primary hepatic carcinomas, a variety of lesions are frequently found in the liver. Common lesions such as hepatic hemangioma, focal nodular hyperplasia, and metastatic disease are well known to clinicians and have been extensively documented in the literature. However, in centers with highly active liver surgery programs, other rare neoplastic and tumor-like conditions can be seen. It is important to understand these conditions in order to guide workup and differentiate management from that of primary hepatic malignant conditions.

Angiomyolipoma

Hepatic angiomyolipoma (AML) is a mesenchymal neoplasm that contains varying amounts of three discrete histologic elements: smooth muscle cells, blood vessels, and adipose tissue [1]. Although the presence of these three elements is considered central to the diagnosis of AML, the varying content of these components can create some diagnostic uncertainty. In fact, the lipid content seen in pathologic specimens has been reported to vary widely, which has led some researchers to subcategorize hepatic AML into four different types based on lines of differentiation and dominant tissue component: mixed, lipomatous (>70% fat), myomatous (<10% fat), and angiomatous [1,2]. However, modern immunohistochemical techniques have markedly increased lesion specificity through positive staining for HMB-45 myoid cells [3].

    Demographically, there appears to be a striking female predominance (5:1 ratio vs. males) with a mean age at diagnosis of 48 years in one study [1]. Although vague symptoms such as epigastric pain, malaise, and weight loss have been described in

Primary Carcinomas of the Liver, ed. Hero K. Hussain and Isaac R. Francis. Published by Cambridge University Press. © Cambridge University Press 2010.

patients with hepatic AML, most patients are asymptomatic [3]. However, as the lesion increases in size, the incidence of symptoms substantially increases. Approximately 20% of patients with lesions less than 5 cm in size will be symptomatic, whereas nearly 90% of patients with lesions greater than 10 cm will demonstrate some symptoms [4]. Hepatic AML is much less common than its renal counterpart, and is more likely to be solitary and sporadic. Only 6% of hepatic AML cases occur in patients with tuberous sclerosis, versus 20% of renal AML cases [5]. Historically, hepatic AML has been thought of as a benign lesion. More recently, there have been extremely rare reports of aggressive and frankly malignant behavior associated with hepatic AML [6]. Furthermore, the variable histologic appearance of hepatic AML can make it difficult to diagnose on fine-needle aspirates, with features that can lead to the erroneous diagnosis of HCC [7]. Therefore, some have advocated surgical management for all symptomatic patients and continued close follow-up of asymptomatic patients [3].

Imaging characteristics of hepatic AML vary with the underlying lesion composition. Ultrasound may demonstrate a highly echogenic lesion with speed propagation and refraction artifact [5]. Computed tomography (CT) generally reveals a predominantly low-density lesion, sometimes with a distinct fat attenuation component and soft tissue attenuation component [2]. With intravenous contrast, rapid enhancement has been reported with a later peak than that of HCC, thought to be related to the highly vascularized nature of the fatty tissue within hepatic AML [5]. Appearance on magnetic resonance imaging (MRI) is directly related to the underlying tissue composition. Hepatic AML composed predominantly of fat will demonstrate features of macroscopic fat on MRI, with high signal intensity on T1-weighted images that nullifies with fat-suppression techniques [5] (Figure 12.1). Areas containing multiple elements will demonstrate signal loss on opposed-phase gradient-echo imaging versus in-phase imaging, indicative of the signal cancellation between adipocytes and non-fatty elements in a voxel [8] (Figure 12.1a–b). Hepatic AML often has a heterogeneous appearance on T2-weighted imaging with predominantly increased signal intensity versus background parenchyma due to fat content that nullifies with fat suppression or on short-tau inversion recovery (STIR) images (Figure 12.1c), and variable enhancement on postcontrast T1-weighted imaging (Figure 12.1d) [9]. Lesions with minimal fat content will have nonspecific imaging characteristics on all modalities, and could mimic HCC (Figure 12.2, a–d) [8]. Therefore, tissue confirmation would be required in patients who desire conservative management.

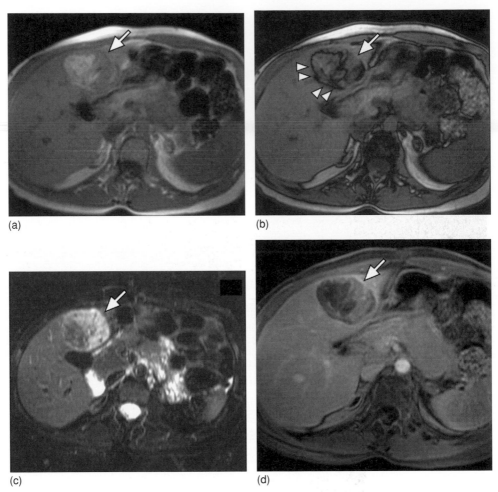

(a)　　　　　　　　　　　(b)

(c)　　　　　　　　　　　(d)

Figure 12.1 (a–d): Hepatic AML (*arrow*) in the medial segment of the left lobe (IV). Axial in-phase T1-weighted gradient-echo MR image (a) demonstrates the heterogeneous increased signal intensity (*arrow*) of the mass versus background hepatic parenchyma due to the presence of lipid and fat. Axial opposed-phase T1-weighted gradient-echo MR image (b) demonstrates visual loss of signal in the lesion, corresponding to the areas of high signal intensity on matched in-phase T1-weighted image at the same level and indicating the presence of lipid. There is phase cancellation artifact seen as a curvilinear very low signal around several areas of this lesion (*arrowheads*), indicative of an interface between protons of fat within the lesion and water in adjacent liver. (c): Axial short-tau inversion recovery (STIR) MR image demonstrates heterogeneous high signal within the lesion (*arrow*) due to nulling of fat. (d): Axial post-gadolinium T1-weighed gradient-echo MR image demonstrates heterogeneous enhancement within the lesion (*arrow*). The imaging features are characteristic of a hepatic AML, which was subsequently proven on core biopsy.

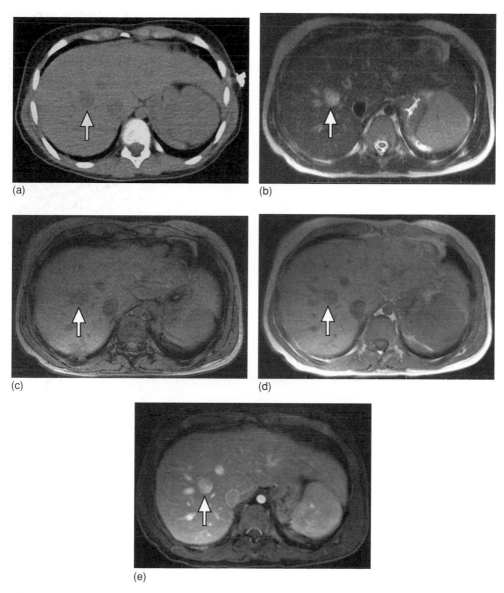

(a)

(b)

(c)

(d)

(e)

Figure 12.2 (a–e): Lipid-poor AML (*arrow*) in segment VIII of the right lobe. (a): Axial noncontrast CT image demonstrates a lesion in the right hepatic lobe, with low internal attenuation versus background hepatic parenchyma. (b): Axial T2-weighted single shot fast-spin-echo MR image shows heterogeneous increased fat signal within the lesion (*arrow*). (c): Axial opposed-phase T1-weighted gradient-echo MR image shows the lesion (*arrow*) with no substantial visual loss of signal within the lesion or at its interface with hepatic parenchyma. This was confirmed by quantitative measurements. (d): Axial in-phase T1-weighted gradient-echo MR image demonstrates a concordant lesion (*arrow*) versus the prior CT study, with low signal intensity versus background hepatic parenchyma. (e): Axial postgadolinium T1-weighed gradient-echo MR image demonstrates contrast enhancement within the lesion (*arrow*). Several biopsy samples were obtained, demonstrating a lipid-poor AML, which had a positive immunohistochemical stain for HMB-45.

Lipoma

True hepatic lipomas are rare lesions, even more uncommon than hepatic AML [10]. Histologically, lipomas are nonencapsulated lesions that are composed entirely of mature adipose tissue [8]. Imaging features are only sparsely described given the rarity of the lesions. On ultrasound, the lesions are usually well circumscribed and highly echogenic [5]. On both CT and MRI, hepatic lipomas will demonstrate characteristics of macroscopic fat. For CT, this includes a well-circumscribed lesion with homogeneous fat attenuation, and a paucity of enhancement on postcontrast images [2]. On MRI, the lesion will demonstrate uniform increased signal intensity on T1-weighted images with phase-cancellation artifact on opposed-phase imaging at the interface of the lesion with adjacent hepatic parenchyma due to the coexistence of fat and water within the same voxels, complete nullification of signal on fat-suppressed imaging, and no substantial enhancement on postgadolinium images [2,8]. It is important to recognize that a lipomatous or lipid-rich hepatic AML (Figure 12.3, a–f) can have identical imaging characteristics to a true hepatic lipoma. In fact, the two lesions may require immunohistochemical staining for accurate differentiation.

Inflammatory pseudotumor

Inflammatory pseudotumor (IPT) (Figure 12.4) is an uncommon liver lesion that is characterized by chronic inflammation and fibroblast proliferation [11]. These lesions occur throughout the body, but are most commonly encountered in the lung; the liver represents the second most commonly affected site [12]. Grossly, these lesions are encapsulated, firm masses. Histologic features include polyclonal plasma cell infiltrates and a dense fibrous stroma, with a characteristic whorled appearance [11,13,14]. The exact etiology and pathogenesis is uncertain, but an infectious cause has emerged as the leading proposed etiology, even though most pathology specimens harbor no objective proof of microorganisms [15]. Some histologic features overlap with the peribiliary changes seen in recurrent pyogenic cholangitis, leading some researchers to suggest a link between the two conditions [14]. The majority of patients will demonstrate nonspecific symptoms such as fever, abdominal pain, or weight loss. Jaundice may result if the lesion is located near the biliary tree. Frequently, leukocytosis and elevated erythrocyte sedimentation rate will be seen on laboratory analysis [11]. Elevation of the cancer antigen (CA) 19–9 tumor marker has also been reported [12]. The prognosis for IPT

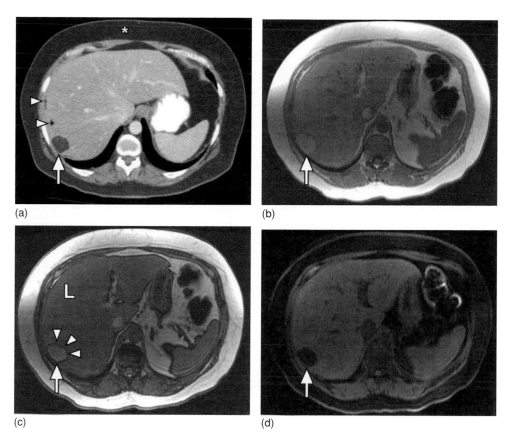

Figure 12.3 (a–f): Lipid-rich AML (*arrow*) mimicking a lipoma in segment VII of the liver. (a): Axial contrast-enhanced CT image demonstrates a lesion in the posterior right hepatic lobe (*arrow*) with very low attenuation versus background hepatic parenchyma. The degree of intralesional low attenuation is visually similar to subcutaneous fat (*asterisk*). Foci of adjacent gas are related to attempted biopsy (*arrowheads*). (b): Axial in-phase T1-weighted gradient-echo MR image demonstrates uniform high signal intensity within the lesion (*arrow*). (c): Axial opposed-phase T1-weighted gradient-echo MR image demonstrates no visual loss of signal within the lesion (*arrow*) versus the in-phase image. There is a prominent rim of signal void, suggesting an interface between protons associated with fat and water (*arrowheads*). Note background loss of signal within the liver parenchyma (L) compatible with hepatic steatosis. (d): Axial fat-suppressed pregadolinium T1-weighted gradient-echo MR image demonstrates near uniform loss of signal within the lesion (*arrow*) as compared to (b) with spectral fat suppression. This finding suggests macroscopic fat. (e): Axial fat-suppressed postgadolinium T1-weighted gradient-echo MR image demonstrates very faint enhancement of several septae within the lesion (*arrow*). There is an overall paucity of solid enhancement. The patient underwent wedge resection of the lesion. (f): Gross histopathologic specimen photograph demonstrates the lesion (*arrow*). Initial biopsies performed at an outside hospital revealed a diagnosis of hepatic lipoma. Because of persistent right upper quadrant discomfort and the patient's desire for surgical management, the lesion was removed via laparoscopy. Although the macroscopic features suggest a predominantly fat-containing lesion, immunohistochemical staining was positive for HMB-45, leading to a diagnosis of a lipid-rich AML. (See color plate section.)

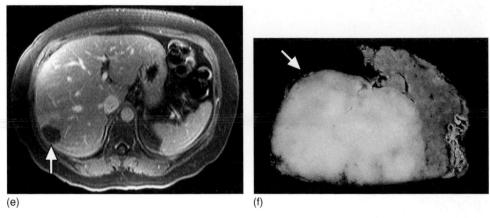

(e)   (f)

Figure 12.3 (*cont.*)

is excellent, with lesion regression seen both spontaneously and following antibiotic therapy [15].

Given the rarity of hepatic IPT, the imaging findings are sparsely discussed and generally nonspecific. Ultrasound usually reveals a heterogeneous lesion with foci of high echogenicity, corresponding to the areas of concentrated fibrosis [16]. CT usually demonstrates a nonspecific mass with increased attenuation versus background hepatic parenchyma on delayed-phase, contrast-enhanced images (Figure 12.4a), particularly in the periphery of the lesion [11]. MRI appearance is also nonspecific, with low signal intensity versus background hepatic parenchyma on T1-weighted images (Figure 12.4b), isointense to mildly hyperintense signal on T2-weighted images (Figure 12.4c), and nonspecific enhancement on postgadolinium imaging (Figure 12.4d) [8]. Unfortunately, the nonspecific imaging appearance necessitates either biopsy or lesion resection for definite histologic characterization. The need for histologic certainty is underscored by the clinical differential diagnosis, which includes intrahepatic cholangiocarcinoma, hepatic abscess, and HCC.

Mesenchymal hamartoma

Although mesenchymal hamartoma is the second most common hepatic mass in children younger than 2 years, it is extremely rare in adults with approximately 20 cases reported in the English literature [17]. Histologically, the lesion is characterized by the presence of several elements, including well-differentiated ductal structures, islands of hepatocytes, and angiomatous elements, plus a surrounding stroma of mature fibroblasts [17,18]. Macroscopically, the lesions in both

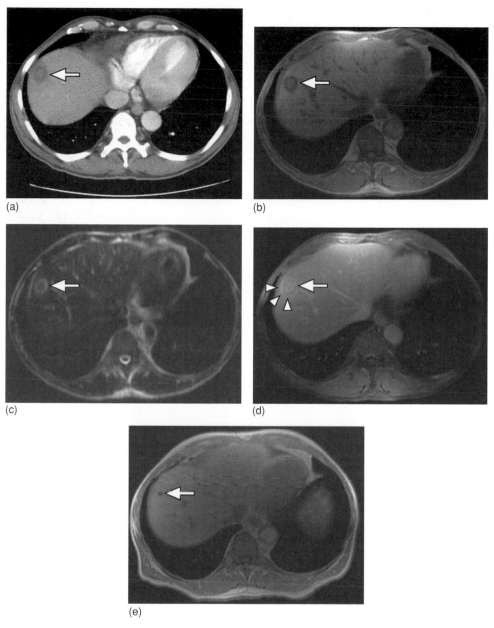

Figure 12.4 (a–e): IPT (*arrow*) in segment VIII of the liver. (a): Axial contrast-enhanced CT image demonstrates a lesion in the right hepatic dome (*arrow*). There is a rim of low attenuation versus background hepatic parenchyma, whereas the central portion is more isoattenuating. (b): Axial in-phase T1-weighted gradient-echo MR image demonstrates the lesion (*arrow*) with a similar morphology to the CT study, including a low-signal-intensity rim and central isointensity. (c): Axial T2-weighted single-shot fast spin echo MR image demonstrates the lesion (*arrow*) with a high-signal-intensity rim and central isointensity. (d): Axial fat-suppressed postgadolinium T1-weighted gradient-echo MR image demonstrates the lesion (*arrow*) with some central intralesional enhancement and a non-enhancing hypointense rim. There is some perilesional hyperintensity (*arrowheads*). Because the MRI features were nonspecific, biopsy was obtained, revealing a diagnosis of IPT. (e): Axial in-phase T1-weighted gradient-echo MR image obtained almost 9 months later than Figure 12.1b. Despite no interval therapy, the lesion (*arrow*) had markedly decreased in size, corroborating the benign nature of an IPT.

children and adults often have a cystic predominance and can grow to massive sizes. They have been reported to occur more frequently in the right lobe than in the left lobe of the liver. Although these lesions are often asymptomatic in childhood, the adult form of mesenchymal hamartoma is associated with abdominal pain in approximately 50% of cases. Various theories about the etiology of these lesions have been proposed, including a developmental abnormality of the ductal plate or reactive change to ischemic injury [18]. Some recent immunohistochemical and flow cytometry analyses have suggested that the stromal component may in fact be a precursor to undifferentiated embryonal sarcoma [19]; there have been no reports of malignant conversion in adults to date. From an imaging perspective, the lesions often have nonspecific features and reflect the varying underlying tissue elements. The cystic spaces of mesenchymal hamartoma show characteristics of simple fluid – namely, anechoic spaces on ultrasound, fluid attenuation on CT, and high signal intensity on T2-weighted MRI [20]. Solid areas manifest as nonspecific intralesional soft tissue on all modalities (Figure 12.5, a–c). Although mesenchymal hamartoma is thought to be a primarily benign lesion, recommended treatment is surgical with the goal of total tumor removal, either via enucleation of the lesion itself or hepatic transplantation if local resection is not technically possible [17].

Biliary hamartoma

Biliary hamartomas are small, benign malformations of the bile ducts that result from incomplete involution of the embryonic bile-duct network [21]. Although they can be found in isolation, biliary hamartomas are often encountered as multiple lesions [22]. Initially described by von Meyenburg in 1918 (and subsequently referred to as von Meyenburg complexes), biliary hamartomas can have a variety of histologic patterns that vary from predominantly solid lesions with narrow bile channels to mostly cystic lesions with prominent bile channels. Most lesions are smaller than 1.5 cm in size. Communication with the intrahepatic biliary tree is a controversial topic, with reports of positive and negative demonstrable communication present in the literature [23]. As a result, some authors have hypothesized that two forms of biliary hamartomas may exist, including one form that communicates with the proper biliary tree and one form that does not [23]. Incidence of multiple biliary hamartomas in autopsy studies has been reported as varying between 0.6 and 2.8% [24]. Although an association with malignancy has been described, no causative relationship has been proven. Generally thought to be asymptomatic, biliary hamartomas can be confused for metastases on imaging, which may

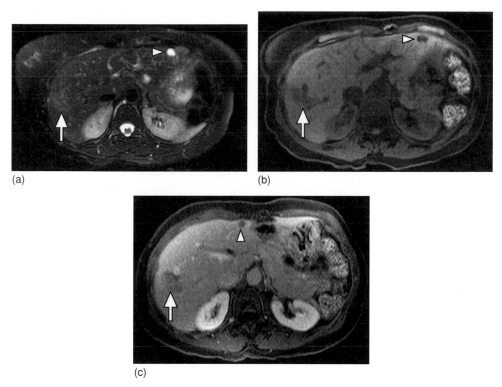

(a)   (b)

(c)

Figure 12.5 (a–c): Mesenchymal hamartoma (*arrow*) in segment VI of the liver. (a): Axial fat-suppressed T2-weighted fast-spin-echo MR image demonstrates an area of subtle signal abnormality (*arrow*), with slightly increased signal intensity versus background hepatic parenchyma. A hepatic cyst is seen in the lateral aspect of the left hepatic lobe (*arrowhead*). (b): Axial fat-suppressed precontrast T1-weighted gradient-echo MR image reveals a geographic area of signal abnormality (*arrow*) that is hypointense versus background hepatic parenchyma. The conspicuity of this area is more pronounced on the T1-weighted image compared to the T2-weighted image, perhaps because the lesion did not contain large cystic spaces. Hepatic cyst is again demonstrated in the lateral segment of the left hepatic lobe (*arrowhead*). (c): Axial fat-suppressed postgadolinium T1-weighted gradient-echo MR image demonstrates some patchy enhancement in the lesion (*arrow*). The findings were nonspecific on MRI, and image-guided biopsy was performed, revealing a diagnosis of mesenchymal hamartoma. An additional hepatic cyst is present in the medial segment of the left hepatic lobe (*arrowhead*).

necessitate biopsy. The imaging appearance across multiple modalities has been described. On ultrasound, a variety of appearances have been cited in the literature, with most lesions described as hypoechoic or anechoic foci that demonstrate posterior acoustic enhancement; hyperechoic foci have been also been reported [21,23]. On CT, biliary hamartomas are seen most frequently encountered as multiple low attenuation foci, most of which demonstrate no internal enhancement

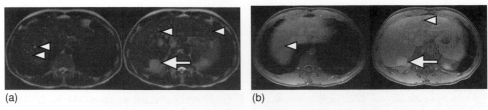

(a)   (b)

Figure 12.6 (a–b): Biliary hamartomas (von Meyenberg complex) (*arrowheads*) throughout the liver. (a): Axial T2-weighted single-shot fast spin-echo MR images demonstrate numerous circular foci of high signal intensity, all less than 1 cm in size (*arrowheads*). A larger focus of signal abnormality in the posterior segment of the right hepatic lobe represents a hemangioma (*arrow*). (b): Axial fat-suppressed postgadolinium T1-weighted gradient-echo MR images demonstrate many foci of low signal intensity versus the enhancing background hepatic parenchyma (*arrowheads*). No solid enhancement within these lesions was reliably demonstrated. Note complete delayed fill of the hepatic hemangioma in the right hepatic lobe (*arrow*).

[22,23]. Rare examples in the literature of enhancement with iodinated contrast have been reported [25]. MRI is considered the best imaging modality for evaluating biliary hamartomas, typically demonstrating low signal intensity on precontrast T1-weighted images and high signal intensity on T2-weighted images, including long echo-time pulse sequences or "heavily T2-weighted sequences" (Figure 12.6 a) [21,26]. Contrast enhancement with gadolinium-based agents on MRI has been variably reported, with many series to date reporting no intralesional enhancement (Figure 12.6b) [23]. More recent studies have demonstrated rim enhancement (thought to represent compressed hepatic parenchyma) or enhancement of a mural nodule, which may relate to the underlying histologic composition [21,26]. Magnetic resonance cholangiopancreatography (MRCP) has demonstrated promise in delineating the periductal nature of biliary hamartomas and separating them from dilated intrahepatic biliary radicals as would be seen in Caroli's disease [21]. Recognition of these imaging features, particularly the MRI appearance, may suggest the correct diagnosis, which can obviate the need for tissue sampling.

Hepatic epithelioid hemangioendothelioma

Hepatic epithelioid hemangioendothelioma (HEH) is a rare lesion composed of epithelioid or dendritic cells that grow along vascular channels (either preformed or neovascular), with a background fibrous and myxohyaline stroma [20]. It is considered a low- to intermediate-grade malignancy, with reported cases of extrahepatic spread to abdominal lymph nodes, the peritoneal surface, and the lungs [27]. Clinical findings are often nonspecific, including right upper quadrant

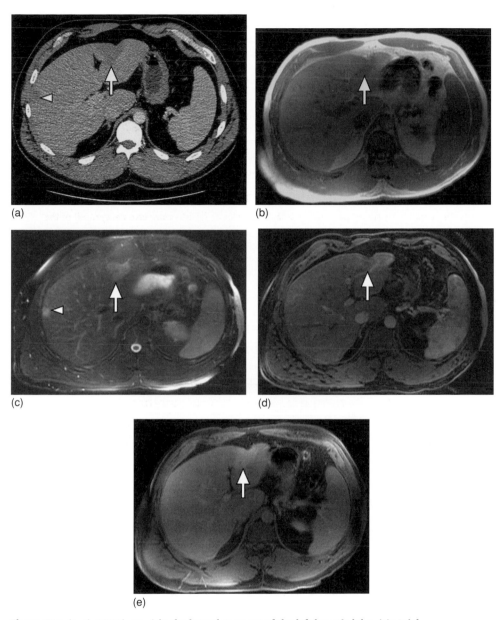

(a)

(b)

(c)

(d)

(e)

Figure 12.7 (a–e): HEH (*arrow*) in the lateral segment of the left hepatic lobe. (a): Axial contrast-enhanced CT image demonstrates a confluent area of low attenuation (*arrow*) in the left hepatic lobe versus background hepatic parenchyma. Note overlying hepatic capsular retraction. An additional lesion is present in the right hepatic lobe (*arrowhead*). (b): Axial in-phase T1-weighted gradient-echo MR image demonstrates a concordant signal abnormality versus the CT study, with low signal intensity versus background hepatic parenchyma (*arrow*). The second lesion seen on CT in the right hepatic lobe was seen on a separate slice of the sequence (not shown). (c): Axial fat-suppressed T2-weighted fast spin-echo MR image demonstrates the lesion (*arrow*) with high signal intensity pain and weight loss. Rarely, a patient can present with fulminant liver failure or Budd–Chiari syndrome [28]. There are two general varieties of HEH: a multifocal form and a diffuse form. The process is believed to originate as multifocal disease that has a characteristic pattern of coalescent growth over time, where multifocal disease evolves temporally into regional or diffuse disease [28]. It is important to distinguish this lesion from other multifocal or diffuse hepatic processes, including metastases, multifocal HCC, or angiosarcoma, as the prognosis for HEH is significantly better than these other differential considerations. Recent immuno-histochemical work has increased diagnostic certainty on pathologic specimens, as HEH tends to stain positive for at least one endothelial marker (factor VIII–related antigen, CD34, or CD31). A variety of treatment options exist for patients with HEH, including orthotopic liver transplantation (even in the setting of known metastases), radiation therapy, or chemotherapy.

From an imaging standpoint, HEH has few specific features. On ultrasound, the multifocal form of HEH is typically seen as multifocal hepatic masses. Although a variety of internal echotextures have been reported, the lesions are generally hypoechoic versus background hepatic parenchyma [28]. Geographical heterogeneous liver echotexture is seen in the diffuse form of HEH. On CT, HEH can appear as multiple hypodense masses or confluent regions, depending on the type of disease. Peripheral location of the lesions is characteristic (Figure 12.7a), often with extension to the capsular surface, although the presence of frank capsular retraction due to intralesional fibrosis is estimated to be only 25% (Figure 12.7) [20]. Some lesions will demonstrate central calcification. On contrast-enhanced CT imaging, arterial-phase marginal enhancement has been noted, with subsequent decreased conspicuity versus enhancing parenchyma on venous-phase imaging [28]. MRI features have also been reported, including low signal intensity on precontrast T1-weighted images versus background hepatic parenchyma (Figure 12.7b) and

Figure 12.7 (*cont.*) versus background hepatic parenchyma. The second lesion on CT is seen in the right hepatic lobe in this series (*arrowhead*). (d): Axial fat-suppressed postgadolinium T1-weighted gradient-echo MR image obtained during the late arterial phase of enhancement demonstrates only minimal patchy internal enhancement of the dominant lesion in the left hepatic lobe (*arrow*). The second lesion in the right hepatic lobe was present on a separate slice of this sequence (not shown). (e): Axial fat-suppressed postgadolinium T1-weighted MR image obtained several minutes after contrast administration demonstrates retention of contrast material within the lesion (*arrow*). The second lesion in the right hepatic lobe was present on a separate slice of this sequence (not shown), and also demonstrated delayed enhancement. Subsequent biopsy of the dominant lesion demonstrated HEH.

heterogeneous increased signal intensity on T2-weighed images (Figure 12.7c). A target appearance of these lesions on T2-weighted sequences has been described, with central areas of low signal intensity on T2-weighted images attributed to central hemorrhage, coagulative necrosis, or calcification [20]. Recently, one group has described a peripheral ringlike appearance with several rims that have increased signal intensity on T1-weighted images and very low signal intensity on T2-weighted images, postulated to be accumulated proteinaceous and ferrous debris in thrombosed vascular channels [29]. The lesions often demonstrate peripheral enhancement upon intravenous gadolinium contrast administration (Figure 12.7d) with intense delayed enhancement (Figure 12.7e). Although the correct diagnosis may be confidently suggested in the setting of multifocal peripheral lesions (with associated capsular retraction) that coalesce on serial examinations, specific findings are rarely present on a single-time-point examination. Therefore, tissue sampling is often required to confidently establish the diagnosis.

Biliary cystadenoma

Biliary cystadenomas are rare cystic lesions that originate from the hepatobiliary epithelium and often present as large intrahepatic cystic masses [30]. Although they are technically benign lesions, there is a risk of malignant degeneration. The etiology of biliary cystadenoma and its malignant counterpart cystadenocarcinoma is not well understood, but theorized to develop from remnant primitive hepatobiliary tissue [31]. Biliary cystadenomas are almost exclusively lesions of the intrahepatic biliary tree, with increased reported occurrence in the right hepatic lobe. Most patients are females, often middle aged. Clinical features may include non-specific chronic abdominal pain, elevated liver function tests, or even jaundice from mass effect on the biliary tree. Histologically, the lesions are characterized as cystic spaces lined by cuboid or columnar epithelium. Some lesions demonstrate a closely bound stroma of spindle cells that resembles ovarian stroma and has been reported as a pathologic feature favoring benignity [32]. From an imaging standpoint, the lesions appear as non-specific large cystic lesions on all modalities, including ultrasound, CT, and MRI. The lesions are usually multilocular with numerous septae, and often greater than 10 cm in size (Figure 12.8) [32]. The presence of soft tissue nodules has been described on all imaging modalities and is suggestive of malignancy [32]. On MRI, the internal fluid content can manifest as varying signal intensity on precontrast T1-weighted images due to the proteinaceous content of the cyst fluid. Septae and mural nodules should enhance on postcontrast CT or MRI.

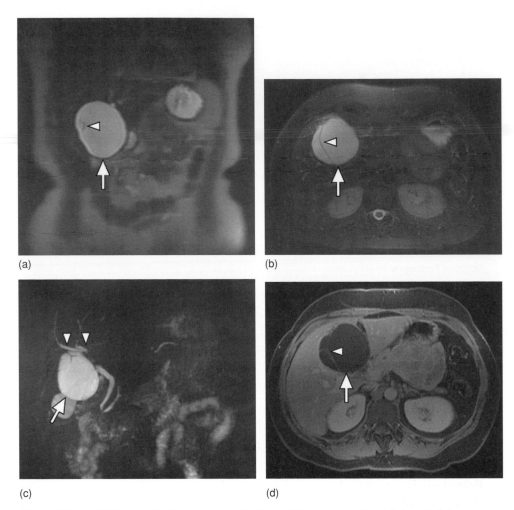

(a)

(b)

(c)

(d)

Figure 12.8 (a–d): Biliary cystadenoma (*arrow*) in the medial segment of the left hepatic lobe (segment IV). (a): Coronal T2-weighted single-shot fast spin-echo MR image demonstrates a large lesion (*arrow*) toward the junction of the right and left hepatic lobes. The lesion demonstrates high signal intensity versus background hepatic parenchyma. There is a prominent septum (*arrowhead*). (b): Axial fat-suppressed T2-weighted fast spin-echo MR image demonstrates the lesion (*arrow*) with prominent septa (*arrowhead*). The lesion measured more than 8 cm in greatest dimension. (c): Maximum intensity projection image generated from a three-dimensional T2-weighted fast-recovery fast spin-echo MRCP sequence demonstrating the lesion (*arrow*), which is exerting mass effect on the central bile ducts, resulting in intrahepatic biliary ductal dilation (*arrowhead*). (d): Axial fat-suppressed postgadolinium T1-weighted gradient-echo MR image demonstrates no dominant solid internal enhancement within the lesion (*arrow*). The thin septum does enhance after gadolinium intravenous contrast administration (*arrowhead*). The patient underwent surgical resection of the lesion, which was found to be a biliary cystadenoma on pathology examination.

MRCP has been reported as valuable in delineating biliary anatomy prior to surgery (Figure 12.8), particularly in cases of segmental biliary obstruction from mass effect [30]. The recommended therapy for both biliary cystadenoma and cystadenocarcinoma is complete surgical resection, which decreases the importance of preoperative discrimination between these two entities [30].

REFERENCES

1. Tsui WM, Colombari R, Portmann BC, *et al.* Hepatic angiomyolipoma: A clinicopathologic study of 30 cases and delineation of unusual morphologic variants. *Am J Surg Pathol* 1999; **23**(1): 34–48.

2. Basaran C, Karcaaltincaba M, Akata D, *et al.* Fat-containing lesions of the liver: Cross-sectional imaging findings with emphasis on MRI. *AJR Am J Roentgenol* 2005; **184**(4): 1103–10.

3. Yang CY, Ho MC, Jeng YM, Hu RH, Wu YM, and Lee PH. Management of hepatic angiomyolipoma. *J Gastrointest Surg* 2007; **11**(4): 452–7.

4. Nonomura A, Mizukami Y, and Kadoya M. Angiomyolipoma of the liver: A collective review. *J Gastroenterol* 1994; **29**: 95–105.

5. Prasad SR, Wang H, Rosas H, *et al.* Fat-containing lesions of the liver: Radiologic-pathologic correlation. *RadioGraphics* 2005; **25**(2): 321–31.

6. Nonomura A, Enomoto Y, Takeda M, *et al.* Invasive growth of hepatic angiomyolipoma; a hitherto unreported ominous histological feature. *Histopathology* 2006; **48**(7): 831–5.

7. Zhong DR and Ji XL. Hepatic angiomyolipoma-misdiagnosis as hepatocellular carcinoma: A report of 14 cases. *World J Gastroenterol* 2000; **6**: 608–12.

8. Fisher A and Siegelman ES. Body MR Techniques and MR of the Liver. In: Body MRI, 1st edn. Philadelphia: Elsevier, 2005: 1–62.

9. De Bruecker Y, Ballaux F, Allewaert S, *et al.* Solitary hepatic lesion: MRI-pathological correlation of an hepatic angiomyolipoma. *Eur Radiol* 2004; **14**(7): 1324–6.

10. Braga L, Semelka RC, and Armao D. Liver. In: Abdominal-Pelvic MRI, 2nd edn. Hoboken, NJ: Wiley, 2006: 47–447.

11. Fukuya T, Honda H, Matsumata T, *et al.* Diagnosis of inflammatory pseudotumor of the liver: Value of CT. *AJR Am J Roentgenol* 1994; **163**(5): 1087–91.

12. Ogawa T, Yokoi H, and Kawarada Y. A case of inflammatory pseudotumor of the liver causing elevated serum CA19–9 levels. *Am J Gastroenterol* 1998; **93**(12): 2551–5.

13. Zamir D, Jarchowsky J, Singer C, *et al.* Inflammatory pseudotumor of the liver–a rare entity and a diagnostic challenge. *Am J Gastroenterol* 1998; **93**(9): 1538–40.

14. Yoon KH, Ha HK, Lee JS, *et al.* Inflammatory pseudotumor of the liver in patients with recurrent pyogenic cholangitis: CT-histopathologic correlation. *Radiology* 1999; **211**(2): 373–9.

15. Tsou YK, Lin CJ, Liu NJ, Lin CC, Lin CH, and Lin SM. Inflammatory pseudotumor of the liver: Report of eight cases, including three unusual cases, and a literature review. *J Gastroenterol Hepatol* 2007; **22**(12): 2143–7.

16. Nam KJ, Kang HK, and Lim JH. Inflammatory pseudotumor of the liver: CT and sonographic findings. *AJR Am J Roentgenol* 1996; **167**(2): 485–7.

17. Hernández JC, Alfonso C, González L, *et al.* Solid mesenchymal hamartoma in an adult: A case report. *J Clin Pathol* 2006; **59**(5): 542–5.

18. Yesim G, Gupse T, Zafer U, and Ahmet A. Mesenchymal hamartoma of the liver in adulthood: Immunohistochemical profiles, clinical and histopathological features in two patients. *J Hepatobiliary Pancreat Surg* 2005; **12**(6): 502–7.

19. Bove KE, Blough RI, and Soukup S. Third report of t(19q)(13,4) in mesenchymal hamartoma of liver with comments on link to embryonal sarcoma. *Pediatr Dev Pathol* 1998; **1**: 438–42.

20. Kim KA, Kim KW, Park SH, *et al.* Unusual mesenchymal liver tumors in adults: Radiologic-pathologic correlation. *AJR Am J Roentgenol* 2006; **187**(5): W481–9.

21. Mortelé B, Mortelé K, Seynaeve P, Vandevelde D, Kunnen M, and Ros PR. Hepatic bile duct hamartomas (von Meyenburg complexes): MR and MR cholangiography findings. *J Comput Assist Tomogr* 2002; **26**(3): 438–43.

22. Lev-Toaff AS, Bach AM, Wechsler RJ, Hilpert PL, Gatalica Z, and Rubin R. The radiologic and pathologic spectrum of biliary hamartomas. *AJR Am J Roentgenol* 1995; **165**(2): 309–13.

23. Wohlgemuth WA, Böttger J, and Bohndorf K. MRI, CT, US and ERCP in the evaluation of bile duct hamartomas (von Meyenburg complex): A case report. *Eur Radiol* 1998; **8**(9): 1623–6.

24. Maher MM, Dervan P, Keogh B, and Murray JG. Bile duct hamartomas (von Meyenburg complexes): Value of MR imaging in diagnosis. *Abdom Imaging* 1999; **24**(2): 171–3.

25. Martinoli C, Cittadini G, Jr., Rollandi GA, and Conzi R. Case report: Imaging of bile duct hamartomas. *Clin Radiol* 1992; **43**: 203–5.

26. Tohmé-Noun C, Cazals D, Noun R, Menassa L, Valla D, and Vilgrain V. Multiple biliary hamartomas: Magnetic resonance features with histopathologic correlation. *Eur Radiol* 2008; **18**(3): 493–9.

27. Makhlouf HR, Ishak KG, and Goodman ZD. Epithelioid hemangioendothelioma of the liver: A clinicopathologic study of 137 cases. *Cancer* 1999; **85**(3): 562–82.

28. Lyburn ID, Torreggiani WC, Harris AC, *et al.* Hepatic epithelioid hemangioendothelioma: Sonographic, CT, and MR imaging appearances. *AJR Am J Roentgenol* 2003; **180**(5): 1359–64.

29. Economopoulos N, Kelekis NL, Argentos S, *et al.* Bright-dark ring sign in MR imaging of hepatic epithelioid hemangioendothelioma. *J Magn Reson Imaging* 2008; **27**(4): 908–12.

30. Lewin M, Mourra N, Honigman I, *et al.* Assessment of MRI and MRCP in diagnosis of biliary cystadenoma and cystadenocarcinoma. *Eur Radiol* 2006; **16**(2): 407–13.

31. Horton KM, Bluemke DA, Hruban RH, Soyer P, and Fishman EK. CT and MR imaging of benign hepatic and biliary tumors. *RadioGraphics* 1999; **19**(2): 431–51.

32. Buetow PC, Buck JL, Pantongrag-Brown L, *et al.* Biliary cystadenoma and cystadenocarcinoma: Clinical-imaging-pathologic correlations with emphasis on the importance of ovarian stroma. *Radiology* 1995; **196**(3): 805–10.

Index